GOODBYE LUPUS, HELLO DELICIOUS:

Recipes to Reverse Autoimmune Diseases

with Supermarket Foods

WHAT PEOPLE ARE SAYING ABOUT DR. BROOKE GOLDNER:

It was November 18th 2019 that my rheumatologist called me, to advise me, my diet had been contributing to my health and I no longer had to take medication for my lupus and APS. I had started Dr. Goldner's Goodbye Lupus protocol on March 5th, 2019. I advised all my doctors and followers on social media.

Lupus had forced its way into my life in the worst ways imaginable. Just barely 2 months after my beautiful daughter was born, I had suffered multiple strokes. I had a hidden blood clotting disorder called APS attributed, and often linked, with lupus.

I didn't realize I had shown signs of lupus earlier via skin rashes in the sun, I had spent months trying to know what it was. The strokes unfortunately caused post stroke epilepsy.

I was somehow fortunate from one of my seizures to come across Dr. Brooke Goldner. I had suffered a bad injury from one of my recent seizures down a staircase. I was openly talking about lupus on Megyn Kelly's TV show. Dr. Goldner nearly side tackled me afterwards claiming she could reverse my incurable lupus. After another bad seizure and zero hope from the doctors surrounding me, I decided to give Dr. Goldner a call.

So often we diminish food and nutrients, however the power of food is astounding. Dr. Goldner's Rapid Recovery program was by far one of the hardest resets I've ever done. It was testimonials like this that told me it works to help me through it.

Dr. Goldner helped put my very aggressive lupus into remission, and not only that, her protocol helped turn my very scary bloody clotting disorder APS from positive to negative on my blood reports.

I still to this day, everyday, drink my huge green smoothie. I eat vegan and I try to limit obvious junk.

I owe my life to Dr. Goldner! She helped me have the courage to take care of my own body and destiny. Thank you once again for getting rid of my lupus! Do her program BEFORE you suffer the damage!

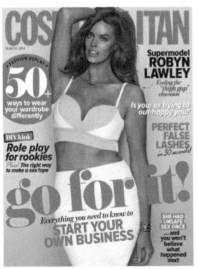

Robyn Lawley
Supermodel
Host of the EveryBody Podcast

Photograph by Kane Skinner

WHAT PEOPLE ARE SAYING ABOUT DR. BROOKE GOLDNER:

Dr. Brooke Goldner has been an important part in helping to educate the community for years. She's kind, personable, and speaks to our viewing audience, as if they were her own family and friends. The information she shares is understandable by anyone, and we take the health of our viewers very seriously. But she also makes it fun! To have the ability to explain complicated, difficult subjects that are very personal, it is difficult for some. But not for her. And that's why the audience likes her and we love it when she visits our show. If she can make eating fruits and vegetables and getting healthy fun, it makes it fun for people to do on a daily basis. Thank you Dr. Goldner for helping our audience get on the right track of health. It is a true benefit in the overall well-being of the viewers we talk to each and every day!

Sharron Melton
News Anchor
CW39 Houston

Dr. Goldner is my go-to for plant-based, disease reversal, recipes, wisdom, and all-around spunk. I have loved interviewing her from Houston to New York and know she provides a wealth of information for all who seek to reverse disease as well as learn more about her plant-based Hyper-nourishment protocol.

I am so happy to see her come out with this recipe book! I told my family last night... "Finally, an easy-to-follow book with all of Dr. Goldner's yummy life saving recipes." And of course, we all nod our heads in approval! Looking at her on social media always makes me want to make the healthy drinks and treats I see her make... now I have the road map to do just that.

I am super excited to have my whole family eating a little healthier... and they don't even know it. I always love it when Dr. Goldner comes on my TV show(s), but now I can take her years of wisdom with me. Just to be clear, I don't know how to cook well, but luckily Dr. Goldner has excellent bedside manner when talking to clients, TV viewers and readers... so I know everyone will love how easy she makes it to prepare these recipes! Thanks Doc!

Shannon Lanier
TV Host -- Houston CW-39, BeWell, Cheddar TV

Any time Dr. Goldner is on our show it is such a great experience. She is kind and caring and always has a smile to share. Dr. Goldner knows first-hand the struggles of a debilitating autoimmune disease and has battled bravely through it. She now shares her story with the world for so many to find answers about their condition and just feel so much better.

Dr. Goldner has made a huge impact on our family. We drink green smoothies almost every day to get the nutrition we need. And we have seen and felt so many benefits from this lifestyle change. Because of her impact on my life, I am so excited to see her new recipe book come to life.

We trust Dr. Goldner all day every day, and really admire the lifesaving work she is able to do through spreading her recipes and protocol to the world.

Sofia Ojeda
KPRC-2 Anchor

Other books by Brooke Goldner, MD

Goodbye Lupus,
How A Medical Doctor Healed Herself Naturally

Goodbye Autoimmune Disease,
How to Prevent & Reverse Chronic Illnesses And Inflammatory Symptoms Using Supermarket
Foods

Green Smoothie Recipes to Kick-Start Your Health & Healing

Published by Plant-Based Health Group LLC, DE

Copyright © 2023 Brooke Goldner, M.D. Houston, TX

Printed in the United States of America First Printing December 2023

FOREWORD

Dr. Brooke Goldner is a visionary in the field of plant-based nutrition and a true advocate for those suffering from chronic illnesses. Her work educating people about the benefits of whole food plant based nutrition has been nothing short of transformative, as she has helped countless individuals to halt and even reverse illnesses, most notably lupus, through her guidance and expertise.

Dr. Goldner's passion for helping others is unwavering, and she has dedicated her life to spreading the message of the power of whole food plant based nutrition. She is a respected and well-known expert in this field, and her deep understanding and knowledge is combined with a gentle, compassionate nature that has made her a trusted and beloved figure among those who seek her help.

In addition to her work as an educator, Dr. Goldner is also a gifted author. Her writing is both engaging and informative, and provides practical, actionable steps for individuals looking to improve their health and wellbeing. She is a true leader in her field, and her unwavering commitment to her mission is an inspiration to us all.

Dr. Goldner's impact on the world of nutrition and health is immeasurable, and her dedication to helping others is a shining example of what it means to be a compassionate and selfless human being. Her work will continue to make a positive impact on the lives of countless individuals for years to come, and she is a true hero in the world of nutrition and health.

Robbie Lockie
Director & Co-founder Plant Based News

Robbie Lockie, born in Zimbabwe, is a prominent figure in the global vegan movement and a digital media expert. They co-founded Plant Based News, a leading source of vegan news with almost 3 million followers on social media, after transitioning to a plant-based diet in 2013 due to health issues. This shift enlightened them about the plight of farmed animals, turning veganism into a significant aspect of their life. Besides Plant Based News, Lockie also initiated the globally recognized World Plant Milk Day and produced informative videos for animal rights organization Viva!. Through these endeavors, they highlight the benefits of veganism for health, environment, and animal welfare, thereby challenging the traditional narrative.

MESSAGE FROM DR. BROOKE GOLDNER

It has been quite astonishing for me as a medical doctor, a scientist, and a lupus conqueror myself, to witness people who have been sick for years, sometimes decades, come back to life and health within days to weeks on my Goodbye Autoimmune Disease Protocol.

Even after years of witnessing these recoveries every day in my wellness practice, I still get goosebumps when I get the news that another person says "Goodbye Autoimmune Disease!"

Today, I heard from 2 mothers whose children healed from lupus after meeting with me for wellness appointments and personalized nutrition plans. The first message was to let me know that her daughter, who was 9 when we met, has been lupus free for a year after our meeting. The second text was from a mother who only met with me one month ago about her 12-year-old daughter who had lupus nephritis. She just got a new test done, and only one month after our meeting, her daughter's urine test came back negative for blood and protein already. Happy tears filled my eyes as I texted back my congratulations. It never gets less thrilling.

I know what it's like after all. I had stage IV lupus nephritis at 16 years old and it took me 2 years on cyclophosphamide chemotherapy and 60mg of prednisone a day (plus a large handful of other pills) to get my first remission, and I still had protein in my urine during this remission, positive labs for lupus, and experienced arthritis, migraines, and photosensitivity. When I was sick, I learned that remission didn't mean I was healthy, just that I wasn't currently dying from my illness.

12 years later, when I did my Goodbye Lupus protocol, symptoms like arthritis and headaches went away, and my labs went back to normal: no protein in my urine, kidney labs normal, lupus antibodies negative, and the blood clot antibodies that I developed later in medical school were gone too! These labs had been abnormal every single time I was tested, and yet suddenly, and from then on, they were negative and normal. Better yet, I was pain-free, energetic, and felt amazing. It turns out, my body just needed the right nutrition, and it could recover and be healthy.

18 years after changing my diet, I have never had a relapse. It's been 30 years since my original lupus diagnosis and many serious life-threatening flares, including mini-strokes that happened while I was sick, yet, I sit here at 46 years old, healthy, energetic, and fit. I have had 2 healthy pregnancies even though I was told I could never have kids. Life is amazing and I am so grateful.

As difficult as my illness was to live with, every moment I was ever sick is worth it today when I get messages like the ones above. Every life saved, every disease reversed, keeps me motivated and inspired to keep spreading the word and help others get their health back too.

When I first recovered my health in 2005, my husband and I assumed it was an amazing, but temporary remission. After 4 years with no relapse, and then having my first son Solomon without any health problems during or after the pregnancy, my husband Thomas and I realized that the change in my diet had truly given me my health back. We wanted to share this with the world, but we were cautious and wanted to make sure we created a scientific protocol that created the same results in other sick people. So, Thomas and I spent over a year studying the impact of nutrition on cellular repair and the immune system. When we believed we understood the protocol necessary to replicate those results, we tested it for free on volunteers. Only when we could consistently replicate the results, did we bring it to the public. We knew this information was essential for saving lives (and for "saving wives" as my husband reminds me), so we decided to release our full protocol to the public for free.

My practice and reputation grew quickly purely through word of mouth, as chronically ill people recovered their health by using our nutrition protocol. Today, our protocol has saved thousands of people from around the world, including many we have never met, who used our free information to heal. I have been honored to be sought out as an educator to help other doctors and medical students learn how to help their patients optimize their nutrition for recovery. I have taught hundreds of doctors from around the world, from the USA, Canada, Germany, Australia and more. I have also taught medical students in the USA and abroad, invited by future doctors and their professors. My heart is filled with hope that the next generation of doctors will have a recipe for our green smoothies on their prescription pad.

Because of my unmatched results in reversing autoimmune disease, in 2021 I was asked by T. Colin Campbell, author of The China Study[6] and a leader in the science behind the movement towards plant-based eating for human health, to be the sole autoimmune professor for his eCornell Plant-Based Nutrition Certificate Program.

In 2022, I became the first plant-based doctor to join the Forbes Health Advisory board. I am overjoyed to be on the board of a trusted mainstream organization that directly impacts the public.
I am thrilled and humbled by these honors. And yet, what still thrills me the most, is helping each person I meet get their health back, achieve their goals, and go after their dreams. That is still what I do every day.

Hyper-nourishment, intentionally over-dosing in nutrition by eating large amounts of nourishing raw plant foods like greens, cruciferous vegetables, flaxseeds and chia seeds is the key to my Goodbye Lupus and Goodbye Autoimmune Disease protocols. Through years of testing foods and observing recovery rates in thousands of people, we have systemized this nutritional approach for disease reversal into these protocols that optimize your ability to completely and quickly repair damage to cells and organs.

I have tested both raw and cooked foods, and have found the raw foods are necessary to create my consistently high rates of disease reversal. While I have had incredible results reversing diseases in thousands of people worldwide over the years starting with my original protocol in my book Goodbye Lupus,[1] I have continued to refine and optimize our protocol over the past decade with all of our experience working with people daily in our Rapid Recovery programs to optimize recovery speed.

Most of my published results come from my Rapid Recovery programs, where I help people reverse inflammation, pain, and diseases in 4-week one-on-one or 6-week group formats. In these programs, my husband Thomas and I help our clients get the nutrition right, make adjustments for food sensitivities, gastrointestinal issues, heart or kidney problems, optimize their plan based off their progress, troubleshoot any issues, and keep them accountable. However, these programs are not just about optimizing nutrition for the fastest recovery possible, but we also add emotional and lifestyle help to keep people motivated and optimize rapid reversal of disease. In essence, I teach them how to make sure their moods are as anti-inflammatory as their foods. I detail this work in how to overcome anxiety, self-sabotage, food addictions and other inflammatory habits and issues in my book, Goodbye Autoimmune Disease.[2]

At the time I am writing this book, over a thousand people have participated in my Rapid Recovery programs, successfully reversing pain and inflammation, dramatically improving laboratory blood markers, blood pressure, weight, and organ function, and creating abundant energy and vitality. Most of these people are now symptom-free and many of them have reduced or completely eliminated their need for medications. They are healthier, happier, and energetic, and living their lives with renewed hope and optimism.

Hyper-nourishment can be done very simply using green smoothies and we have shared our smoothie recipes for free at SmoothieShred.com. But the biggest request we have gotten is for more recipes beyond the green smoothies to get the nourishment in. While I have a few easy delicious raw meals up my sleeve, I also reached out to my Rapid Recovery graduates and asked them to contribute their favorite recipes. We taste-tested the submissions and included our favorites in the book. Their recipes helped them get their health back and can help you do it too! Feel free to change up the recipes in this book according to your taste. You may want to change out the fruits for your favorites, add some fresh herbs, or switch out vegetables for what you happen to have in your kitchen or what's easier for you to find in your local market. The objective is to have fun and get healthy!

As a medical doctor, I know that the healing power of food is woefully missing from the medical school curriculum, limiting doctors to using medications and surgeries to help people survive. Western medicine is great for saving your life, and I still practice medicine for that reason, but medications can never give you health. I believe we must utilize healing nutrition along with life-saving medications to help people heal and then minimize their need for medications in the future.

My goal is to help everyone take back their health and truly live their lives with vigor. These recipes are a great start to adding raw healthy healing plant foods to your diet.

I wish you the most amazing health and a happy life.

Love,
Brooke Goldner, M.D.
GoodbyeLupus.com

To our sweet Alex

We love and cherish you to eternity.

TABLE OF CONTENTS

INTRODUCTION

The Hyper-Nourishment Protocol for Autoimmune Reversal is an intentional overdose of the foods that supply the nutrients that optimize cellular repair and anti-inflammatory immune function.

The human body is estimated to have about 100 trillion cells. Your cells are largely built from the nutrients you consume. While older generations ate from the Earth and ate fresh foods, most of us, me included, were malnourished as children; fed enormous amounts of dairy, meats, processed foods, sugars, and oil. Children today eat the most inflammatory non-nutritive diets in history, and their health has suffered for it. The Western Diet, also known as the Standard American Diet or SAD diet, has created the greatest level of obesity the world has ever known, while also creating the most malnourished or under-nourished people. Yes, people are both obese and malnourished, and have rampant widespread inflammation in their bodies. Recent research indicates a direct correlation between the rise and spread of the Western Diet and the rise and international spreading of autoimmune diseases in areas of the world where they didn't exist before.[7] Other diseases are on the rise as well, like type II diabetes and colon cancer, both of which are now happening in younger people than ever before in history.[3,4]

While scientists debate how to combat our diets with more medical treatments, they tend to underestimate people's willingness to change their diets and the course of their lives.

Changing my diet from a Western Diet laden with dairy, eggs, and processed foods, to a high raw plant-based diet reversed the Lupus I lived with for 12 years. It gave me back my health, my kidneys, and my ability to have a future, to have children, energy and without the pain of arthritis and migraines. It gave me back the ability to enjoy the sun without rashes and flares, and I can look forward to growing old with my husband. At 16 years old, I was on chemotherapy and 7 oral medications a day just to survive. I am 46 years old at the time I write this book, and I require no medications. I am healthier than most people my age and even younger.

I believe everyone should have the chance to choose to do the same. That is why my husband Thomas Tadlock and I chose to release our protocol to the public for free many years ago: because we believe everyone should have the information they need to save their life, and again as my husband says, to save their wife.

The foods you need to eat to get hyper-nourished are simple and easy to find in the supermarket. And the more nourishing meals you eat, and the less meat, dairy and processed foods you eat, the healthier you will be.

We have always tried to make nutritious eating simple and easy, introducing the Smoothie Solution in 2015; where people can put their high nourishment vegetables, flax or chia, and water in a blender with some fruit and drink their way to better health. This was a major breakthrough that helped us get people who don't like to eat veggies to get their nutrients in through a big smoothie straw.

While our Smoothie Solution has saved thousands of lives over the past dozen years, people have often asked for more ideas for healing meals that use the same ingredients that will stimulate cellular repair and the anti-inflammatory immune response that they need to reverse disease and optimize health. This took me a bit longer, since I am a doctor, not a chef, and I decided to ask my clients who have reversed their diseases on my protocol to contribute their favorite recipes to help you enjoy your nourishing meals. Many of them shared their stories too, hoping to inspire you to take back your health bite by bite the way they did!

We tasted and enjoyed every one of these recipes, and we hope you do too!

PART 1
GETTING STARTED

THE FOODS

When it comes to hyper-nourishment, the goal is to intentionally overdose in the most nutrient-dense foods available that promote cellular repair and stimulate the anti-inflammatory immune system, to reverse chronic inflammation and disease.

The protocol is simple and straightforward.

The key tenants for the nutrition, is to eat the foods with the highest levels of vitamins, minerals, antioxidants and omega-3s, which are raw uncooked cruciferous vegetables, spinach and chard, and flax or chia seeds.

While the foods groups for hyper-nourishment are very simple, these recipes combine them in many different ways that your mouth can find as thrilling as your cells do!

While the fastest and most profound results have come for people eating only these raw foods, many people have experienced disease-reversal incorporating these raw nourishing foods into their diet that still includes cooked plant foods like quinoa, beans cooked vegetables and vegetable soups for example.

Even people who eat inflammatory foods like meat and dairy can benefit from adding these foods. It will provide nutrients their bodies need and can crowd out some of the unhealthy foods as they fill up on the good stuff!

Once you get healthy, keep these foods as a major part of your daily diet so you can maintain optimal health and slower aging! A recent study shows that higher intake of cruciferous vegetables is associated with a reduced risk of all causes of mortality, so eat up![5]

Please note, if you are on a low potassium diet because of kidney failure, you will need to use low histamine vegetables, fruits and omega-3 choices. Please check with your doctor if you are not sure or need guidance for this. You can switch out any vegetables and fruits with options that suit your dietary restrictions.

Also if you have allergies and need low-histamine choices, you can substitute low histamine vegetables, fruits and omega-3 sources in any recipe.

The best thing to do is have some fun with it. Try some new things. You might really love some recipes and decide other are not for you. I have found for most people, myself included, that we only need a few favorite recipes to have a lot of food satisfaction. I hope you find some new favorites here, and get inspired to create some new ones of your own.

THE CHEFS

This book contains recipes from my own kitchen, and from my some from my Rapid Recovery clients from around the world who submitted their favorites to help you enjoy your disease-reversing meals!

While most of my clients stick to smoothies and simple salads to nourish themselves back to health, some have come up with creative and delicious recipes to enjoy the healing process even more.

I asked them to send us their favorites. We taste-tested the submissions and served up the most delicious recipes here in this book! We hope you love them too!

Some of our clients also included their names and their stories of recovery to inspire you to nourish yourself back to health the way they did.

I am proud of my chefs and grateful for their contributions to helping you get your health back.

KITCHEN TOOLS

Most of these recipes require some basic kitchen tools, some include some specialized ones to make things even more exciting!

I recommend you have a good set of knives for chopping up fruits and vegetables.

In addition, a high-powered blender will make smoothies, dressings, and sauces much quicker, easier, and tastier to make. A high-powered blender is a professional grade blender that can handle all the daily use and abuse required for raw food preparation! They tend to be expensive, $300-500, but since you will use it so frequently, it is worth the money if you can get one. You can get discounts on refurbished models. I use a Vitamix blender and even after over 10 years of daily use, multiple times a day, my old machine still works really well. I have only replaced the blade once in all that time. I know there are newer models with fancy options, but even if you get a refurbished one, it will do the job. There are other high powered blenders you can try like Blendtec or other brands available in different countries

If you don't have a high-powered blender, or can't afford one, just use the one you have. You may need to blend longer on a weaker machine, so add more ice and keep going until smooth. If a decent blender isn't possible for you right now, stick with the other meals that don't require blending. Use what you have and make it happen!

I also recommend you get a food processor to save time on all the chopping. These can range from $30 to $100 or more depending on the brand. I have done well with a middle of the road food processor from companies like Cuisinart or KitchenAid. There are newer models coming out all the time with attachments and technology, so go with the one you think you will get the most use out of. I like the ones with big bowls for bulk food preparation, like 13-14 cups. If you like to chop by hand, you can totally do that. A mandolin can also help with beautiful thin slices of vegetables and fruits, and they tend to run anywhere from $20 to $100 depending on the brand.

I use a spiralizer for making noodles out of vegetables. It's a great tool, usually costs $20 to $30 and is fun to use with the kids!

There are also some dehydrator recipes included if you want to try them out. You can buy professional dehydrators like Excalibur which makes many different sizes. I have a 9 tray machine for bulk foods like flax crackers or kale chips.

Nowadays, you can buy machines that serve multiple functions. I recently bought a toaster oven that is also an air fryer and a dehydrator, which makes for a lot more counter space!

PART 2
THE RECIPES

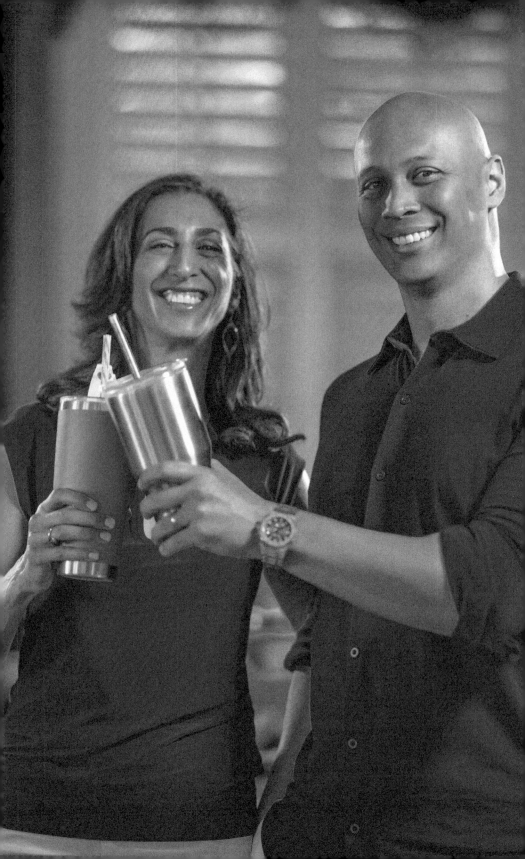

NOURISHING BREAKFAST
& SMOOTHIE RECIPES

So many people begin their day with processed cereals that stimulate the inflammation pathways that cause and exacerbate disease. These delicious recipes are a far better way to start your day!

If you are on the Goodbye Lupus Protocol and Goodbye Autoimmune Disease Protocol, you will most likely want to start your day with a green smoothie made according to my online recipes at SmoothieShred.com. However, here are some additional options if you are looking for something different.

– Brooke Goldner, M.D.

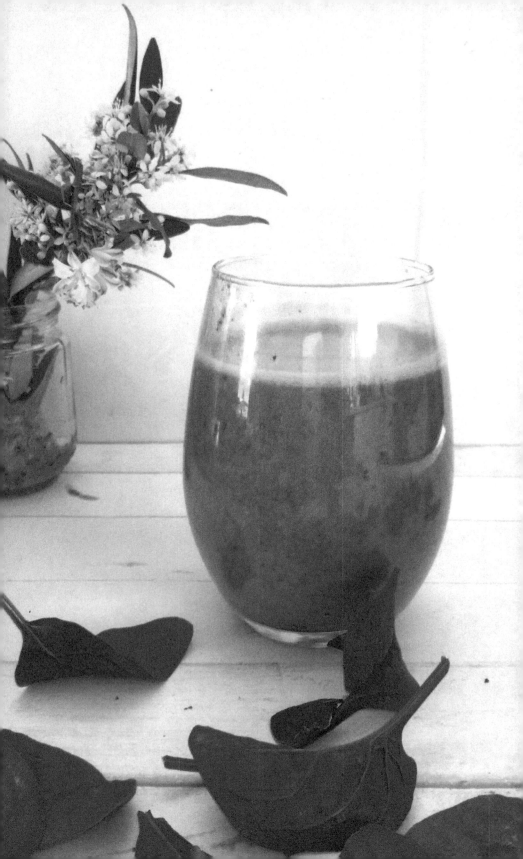

Dr. G's Simple Green Smoothie

Ingredients:

12 oz spinach

3 ripe medium bananas

1 ½ cups frozen mango

4 TB flax seeds

1 cup unsweetened almond milk

Water

Method:

1. Add all the spinach to the blender, making sure to pack it down tightly.

2. Add unsweetened almond milk.

3. Add water until it just covers the spinach.

4. Add all remaining ingredients.

5. Blend for 2-3 minutes on high until liquefied. A low powered blender might need more time.

Recipe note: This recipe is based on using a 64oz or larger high-speed blender. Make sure your fruit is very ripe to deliver full sweetness. Bananas should have brown spots on the skin.

By Brooke Goldner, M.D.

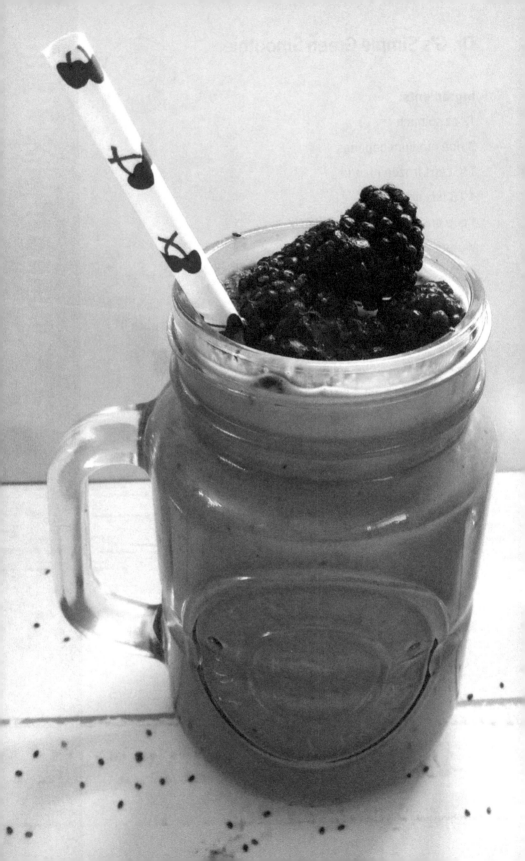

Chocolate Chia Smoothie

Ingredients:

1 cup unsweetened almond milk

3 ½ cups water

1 cup banana

⅓ cup cacao powder

½ cup avocado, frozen

2 TB flax oil

½ cup chia seeds

Method:

1. Place all ingredients in a high-speed blender in the order listed.
2. Blend until smooth.

By Ashley Daniels Lawther

I have psoriatic arthritis. I've had joint pain since I was 8 years old. My disease started getting progressively worse, I was having to double up on my medication and even that was not cutting the pain. Stomach pain attacks would last for about an hour, they were very debilitating, I would sometimes almost pass out from the pain. I couldn't run, I was having difficulty walking, and I was having trouble cooking and doing the dishes. So, I knew I needed to do something different and so I signed up with Dr. Goldner.

Within 30 days my joint pain was significantly better. By the end of the Rapid Recovery program I had no more joint pain. I can run no problem, I have no problem walking. My stomach pain also completely went away. I lost about 10 pounds. My nails are very long and I feel really good. It feels so nice not to just like wake up in the morning and your body feels so good. Like you can move, you can move freely, nothing hurts. I'm so happy I did this and I would definitely recommend this for you all as well.

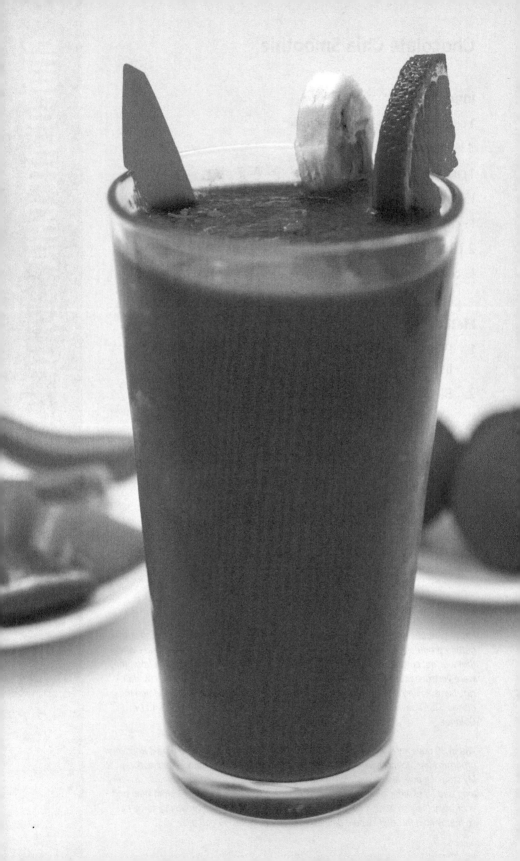

Tropical Trio Smoothie

Ingredients:

32 oz water

12 oz spinach

1 cup banana, frozen

1 cup mango, frozen

1 cup orange, fresh

¼ cup flax or chia seeds

Method:

1. Place all ingredients in a high speed blender in the order listed.
2. Blend until smooth.

Recipe note: *If you'd like to reserve some of your daily fruit allowance to use in a salad or chia pudding, you can use only a half cup of each fruit and this smoothie still tastes great! My favorite version uses sumo citrus for the orange.*

By Julie Teffeteller

In 2018, Julie was diagnosed with undifferentiated connective tissue disease. She suffered from various aches and pains, extreme digestive issues, and generalized anxiety. Following her diagnosis, she spent six months trying to heal through a Paleo/Keto diet and a vast amount of very expensive supplements. While her digestive issues had improved, her pain had significantly increased.

In the summer of 2019, Julie switched to a vegan diet. She ate a lot of fruit, whole grains, and cooked vegetables, but she ate very little greens or healthy fats. She also frequently enjoyed vegan processed foods like rolled oats, rice, pasta, chips, and home baked treats. Her pain levels began to decrease and her digestion issues completely resolved, but she began experiencing significant nervous system issues including high levels of anxiety, tingles, and heart palpitations that woke her in the middle of the night. She was extremely fatigued. She could not work or keep up with her two young boys, and she was afraid to travel too far from home because of her symptoms.

In 2021, Julie enrolled in Dr. Goldner's 4 week one-on-one Rapid Recovery program. Upon completion, she continued the Rapid Recovery protocol on her own after for another4 weeks. After 6 weeks on protocol, her pain had completely disappeared, her energy levels were consistently high all day, and her anxiety had reduced by at least 75%. More importantly, she had the energy to keep up with her boys, and she returned to activities she used to love like going to the beach, visiting theme parks, and boating.

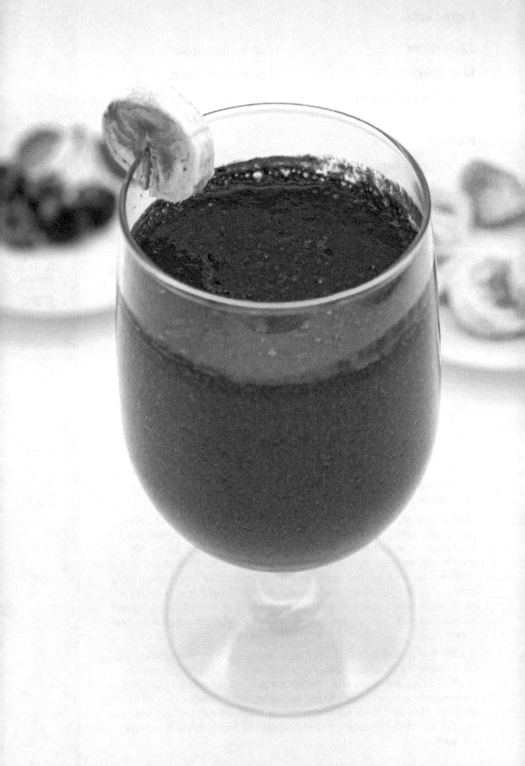

Very Cherry Smoothie

Ingredients:

32 oz water

12 oz spinach

2 bananas, fresh and ripe

2 cups frozen cherry

1-2 TB cacao (optional)

¼ cup flax or chia seed

Method:

1. Place all ingredients in a high-speed blender in the order listed.
2. Blend until smooth.

Recipe note: Adding cacao gives it a chocolate covered cherry spin!

By Julie Teffeteller

In 2018, Julie was diagnosed with undifferentiated connective tissue disease. She suffered from various aches and pains, extreme digestive issues, and generalized anxiety. Following her diagnosis, she spent six months trying to heal through a Paleo/ Keto diet and a vast amount of very expensive supplements. While her digestive issues had improved, her pain had significantly increased.

In the summer of 2019, Julie switched to a vegan diet. She ate a lot of fruit, whole grains, and cooked vegetables, but she ate very little greens or healthy fats. She also frequently enjoyed vegan processed foods like rolled oats, rice, pasta, chips, and home baked treats. Her pain levels began to decrease and her digestion issues completely resolved, but she began experiencing significant nervous system issues including high levels of anxiety, tingles, and heart palpitations that woke her in the middle of the night. She was extremely fatigued. She could not work or keep up with her two young boys, and she was afraid to travel too far from home because of her symptoms.

In 2021, Julie enrolled in Dr. Goldner's 4 week one-on-one Rapid Recovery program. Upon completion, she continued the Rapid Recovery protocol on her own after for another4 weeks. After 6 weeks on protocol, her pain had completely disappeared, her energy levels were consistently high all day, and her anxiety had reduced by at least 75%. More importantly, she had the energy to keep up with her boys, and she returned to activities she used to love like going to the beach, visiting theme parks, and boating.

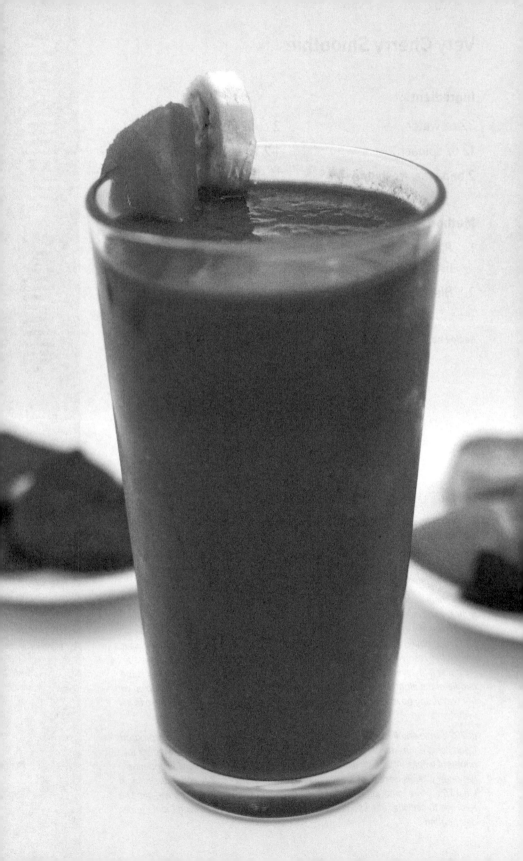

Sunrise Smoothie

Ingredients:

32 oz water

12 oz spinach

½ cup banana, fresh and ripe

½ cup pineapple, frozen

½ cup raspberries, frozen

1 cup mango, frozen

¼ cup flax or chia seed

½ lime, juiced (optional)

Method:

1. Place all ingredients in a high-speed blender in the order listed.

2. Blend until smooth.

By Julie Teffeteller

In 2018, Julie was diagnosed with undifferentiated connective tissue disease. She suffered from various aches and pains, extreme digestive issues, and generalized anxiety. Following her diagnosis, she spent six months trying to heal through a Paleo/ Keto diet and a vast amount of very expensive supplements. While her digestive issues had improved, her pain had significantly increased.

In the summer of 2019, Julie switched to a vegan diet. She ate a lot of fruit, whole grains, and cooked vegetables, but she ate very little greens or healthy fats. She also frequently enjoyed vegan processed foods like rolled oats, rice, pasta, chips, and home baked treats. Her pain levels began to decrease and her digestion issues completely resolved, but she began experiencing significant nervous system issues including high levels of anxiety, tingles, and heart palpitations that woke her in the middle of the night. She was extremely fatigued. She could not work or keep up with her two young boys, and she was afraid to travel too far from home because of her symptoms.

In 2021, Julie enrolled in Dr. Goldner's 4 week one-on-one Rapid Recovery program. Upon completion, she continued the Rapid Recovery protocol on her own after for another4 weeks. After 6 weeks on protocol, her pain had completely disappeared, her energy levels were consistently high all day, and her anxiety had reduced by at least 75%. More importantly, she had the energy to keep up with her boys, and she returned to activities she used to love like going to the beach, visiting theme parks, and boating.

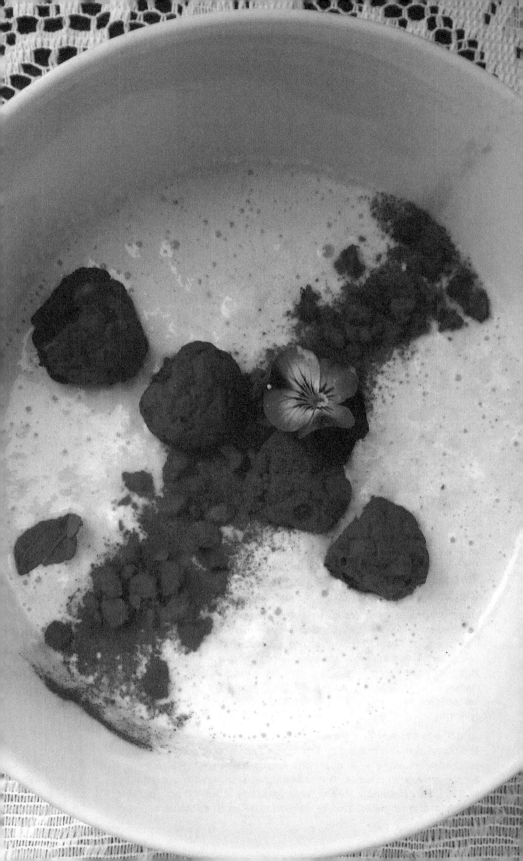

Berry Cauliflower Smoothie

Ingredients:

18 oz cauliflower

1 cup mixed strawberries, blueberries, and bananas

½ cup chia seeds

Mint leaves (optional)

1 tsp maca powder (optional)

1 tsp Ceylon cinnamon

Pinch of cardamom, nutmeg (optional)

Ice cubes (about 5)

Method:

1. Place all ingredients in a high-speed blender in the order listed.
2. Blend until smooth.

By Tina Trtnik

My name is Tina and I was into sports all my life, until a few years ago when inflammation in one knee started to appear for the first time. It got better after steroid injections for a couple of years. But the next time it appeared in both knees, and aspiration and steroids did not help any more. I was pretty much home, resting my legs and missed sports like crazy.

Now that I think back, I can see I had all the signs of autoimmune disease from my teenage years. I had migraines a lot, and they grew more frequent as I aged. I was constipated a lot and nothing helped. I had anxiety and brittle hair. There were numerous signs that my body was not happy and needed help.

I joined Dr. Goldner's 6 Week Rapid Recovery group in May, right before my birthday. I didn't care about anything else, I just wanted my life back. I needed to change everything, not only food, but my outlook on life. I had to learn how to overcome my emotional blockages and learn to think differently, because the life I was living before had driven me to disease.

My knees were pain-free after the group ended, and I kept working on my emotions and food even after I healed. Today I am great. My health has never been better.

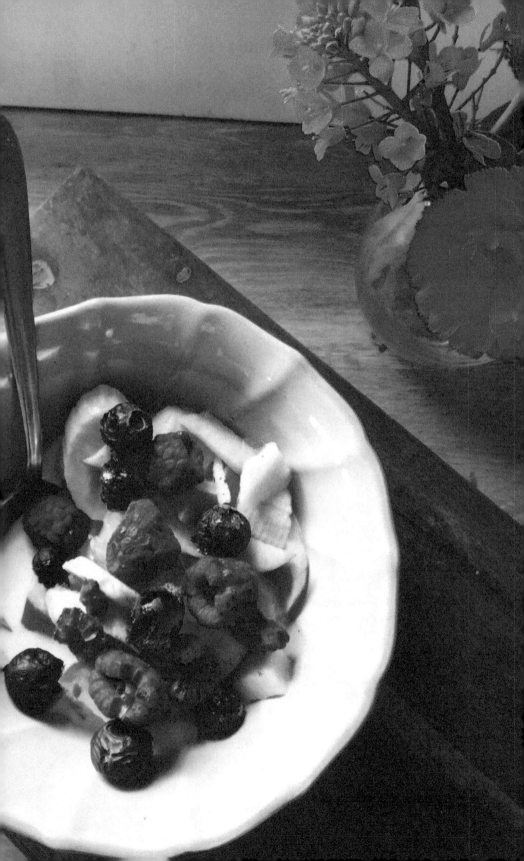

Dr. G's Berry Good Cereal

Ingredients:

1 whole banana sliced

½ cup blueberries, strawberries, (or any berries you like)

¼ cup diced granny smith apples (or any apple you like)

1 cup unsweetened almond milk as desired

Method:

1. Add sliced bananas, berries, or other diced fruits to a bowl.
2. Add unsweetened almond milk until desired level as you would with cold cereal.

By Brooke Goldner, M.D.

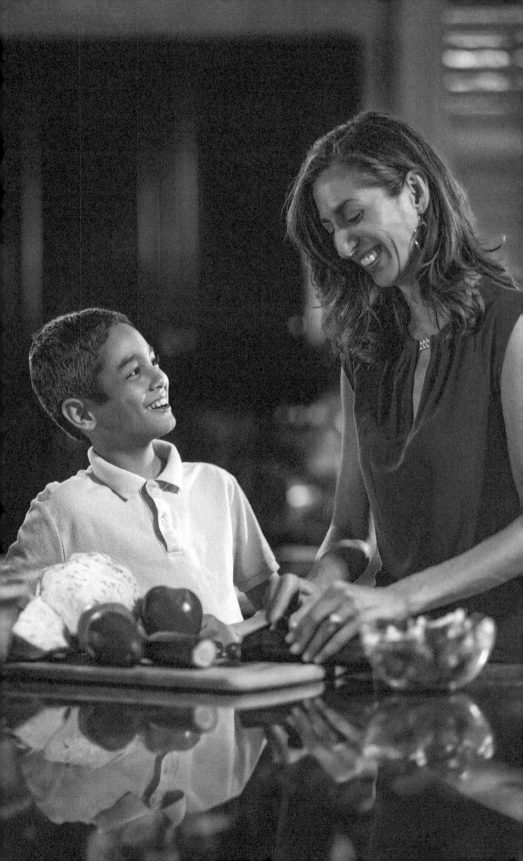

SOUPS &
SALADS

*Healing recipes to satisfy your taste
buds and rev up your metabolism.*

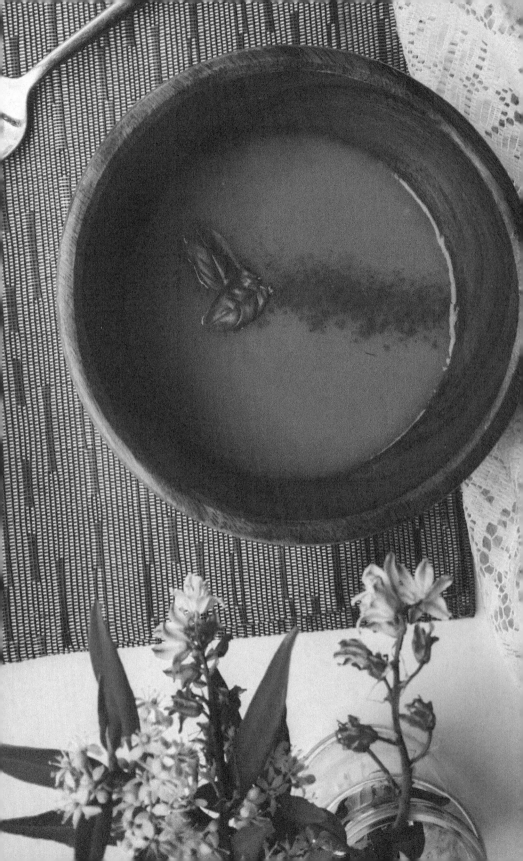

Dr. G's Cold Cantaloupe Soup with a Kick

Ingredients:

1 large cantaloupe melon (cut into chunks for blender)

1 cup cold water

2 TB lime juice

Pinch of chili powder

Pinch of cayenne

Pinch of cinnamon

Method:

1. Place all ingredients in a high-speed blender in the order listed.

2. Blend until smooth.

By Brooke Goldner, M.D.

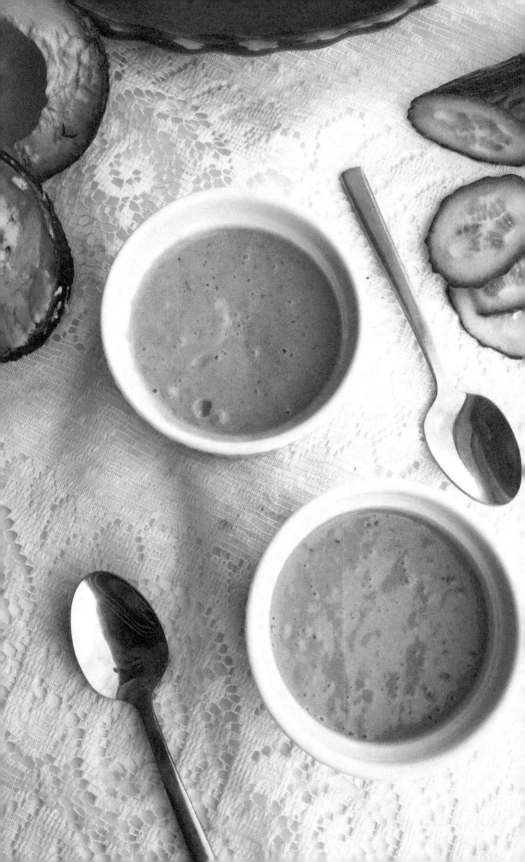

Dr. G's Cold Avocado Cucumber Soup

Ingredients:

16 oz cucumbers

2 small avocados

¼ cup fresh lime juice

¾ cup cold water

1 tsp sea salt (or to taste)

½ tsp black pepper (or to taste)

Method:

1. Blend cucumbers, avocado, and lime juice on high until smooth.

2. Add salt and pepper to taste.

3. Transfer the soup to a large bowl and refrigerate for at least an hour before serving.

By Brooke Goldner, M.D.

Gazpacho Soup

Ingredients:

2 ½ cups ripe red tomatoes

1 small sweet yellow onion

1 cup cucumber, chopped

1 medium red bell pepper, seeded

¼ cup basil

1 garlic clove, peeled

¼ cup ground flaxseeds

2 TB sugar-free red wine vinegar

¼ tsp salt

Ground black pepper to taste

Method:

1. Cut tomato, onion, cucumber, and red bell pepper into 1" chunks.
2. Place all of the onion in a blender.
3. Place half of the tomatoes, cucumber, and red bell pepper into a bowl and the other half into the blender.
4. Add the remaining ingredients to the blender and blend until smooth.
5. Take the rest of the veggies from the bowl and place them in the blender.
6. Pulse until the chunks are smaller but not smooth.
7. Chill gazpacho for at least 2 hours before serving.

By Julie Engelman Kish

Julie was diagnosed with systemic scleroderma, a rare autoimmune disease that causes chronic hardening and tightening of the skin and connective tissues. After Rapid Recovery, Julie continued and still continues the Hyper-nourishment protocol, consuming a pound of greens and a cup of flax in smoothies every day. She is no longer on any medications, feels much more energetic, and her scleroderma has not progressed! She also noted that a bladder issue, which previously caused her to get up 6 or more times per night, was completely healed with the Rapid Recovery protocol!

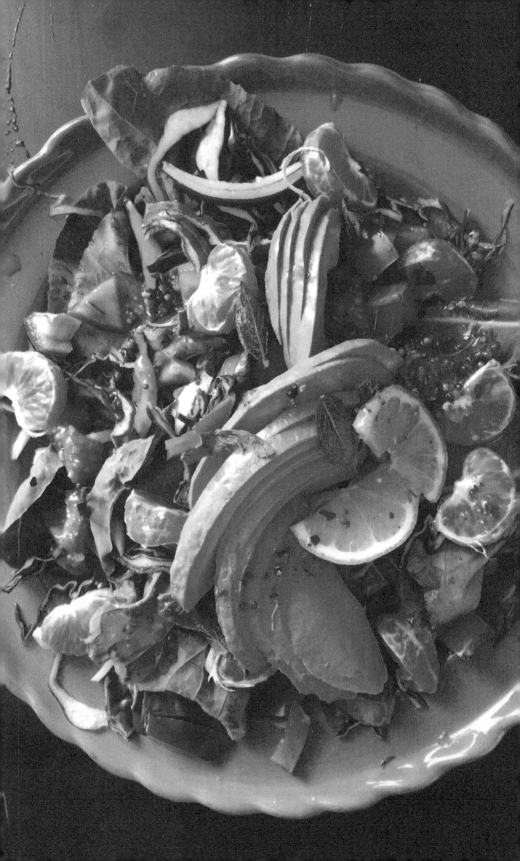

Dr. G's Citrus Cruciferous Salad

Salad Ingredients:

12 oz kale

6 oz red cabbage

1 cup carrot, shredded

½ cup red onion

1 cup Roma tomato, diced

½ cup mandarin oranges

1 ½ cups avocado

Dressing Ingredients:

⅔ cup pineapple

⅔ cup mango

2 TB white vinegar or apple cider vinegar

¼ cup water

1 tsp salt

¼ cup mint

Method:

1. For the dressing, add all the ingredients to a blender and season as desired.

2. Massage some of the Citrus Salad Dressing into the kale and refrigerate about 30 minutes to soften the kale.

3. When you are ready to eat, add rest of ingredients and toss with the rest of the dressing.

By Brooke Goldner, M.D.

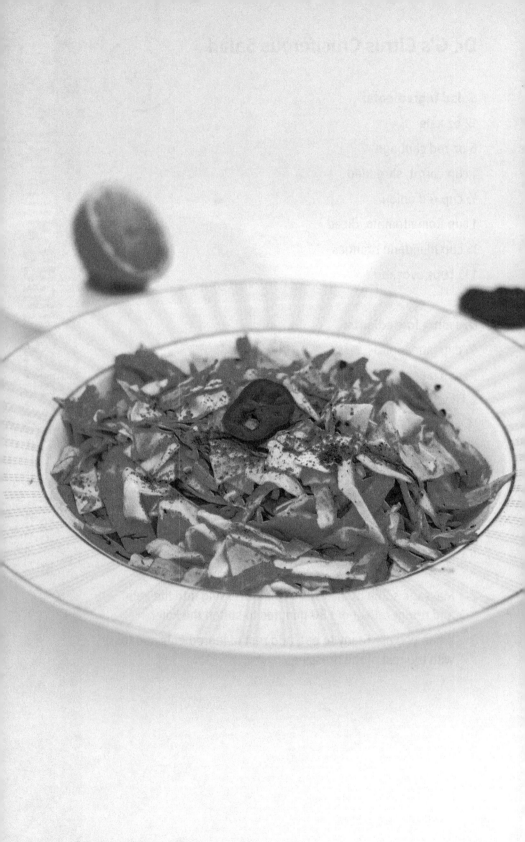

Dr. G's Spicy Cabbage Salad

Ingredients:

12 oz cabbage, chopped

1 TB lemon juice

Dash of cayenne to taste

Salt to taste

1 Tb cold-pressed flaxseed oil (optional)

Method:

1. Combine all ingredients in a bowl and mix well.

Recipe note: Be careful with the cayenne! Start with a little and slowly add more to your taste preference.

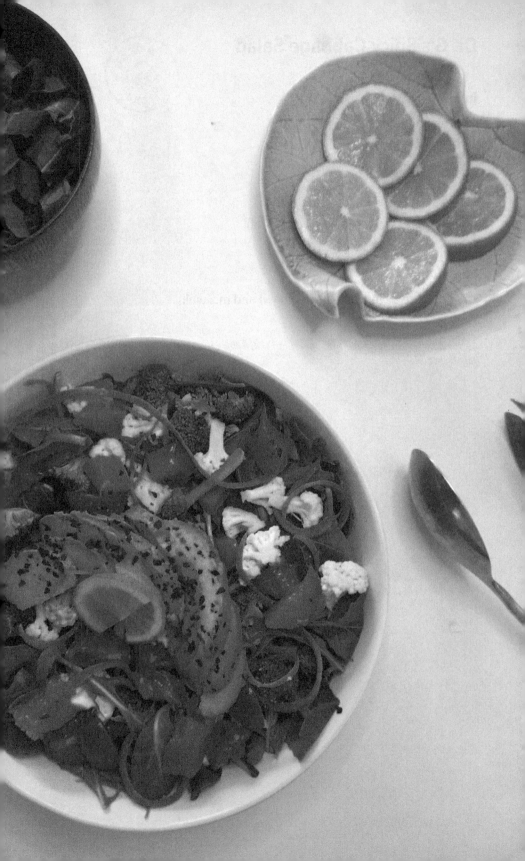

Dr. G's Mango Crunch Salad

Salad Ingredients:

1 cup red or green cabbage

1 cup baby spinach

1 cup tomatoes

1 cup bell pepper

1 cup broccoli

1 cup cauliflower

1 cup cucumbers

1 cup carrots

1 avocado, sliced

¼ cup mango

Dressing Ingredients:

1 TB lemon juice

1 TB Braggs Liquid Aminos

2 TB flaxseed oil

¼ tsp garlic powder

½ tsp salt to taste

Method:

1. Add baby spinach to salad bowl.
2. Slice cabbage into thin slices (or chop if you prefer) and add to salad bowl.
3. Chop the remaining ingredients (except avocado) into bite-sized pieces and add to salad bowl.
4. Blend or whisk dressing ingredients until well combined
5. Pour dressing over the salad and toss.
6. Add sliced avocado on top.

By Brooke Goldner, M.D.

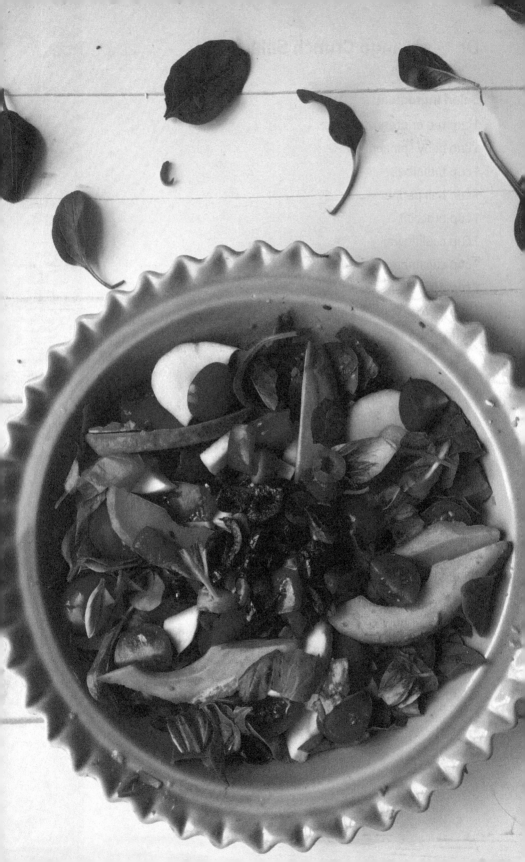

Salad with Olive Tapenade

Tapenade Ingredients:

½ cup olives, chopped

¼ cup red bell pepper, chopped

2 tsp each fresh basil and oregano (or ¼ tsp each dried)

1 tsp garlic, chopped

Salad Ingredients:

4 cups arugula, spinach & radicchio mix, chopped

¼ cup cherry tomatoes, sliced fine

½ cup cremini mushrooms, steamed and sliced

½ avocado for garnish

Method:

1. Combine all tapenade ingredients in a small bowl.
2. In a larger bowl, combine all of the salad ingredients and pour the tapenade over top.

By Fiona Elizabeth

Fiona came to Dr. Brooke Goldner's protocol as a young woman emaciated at 85 pounds, with chronic inflammation and an auto-immune skin condition. Having struggled for many years with her health, she discovered Dr. Goldner's approach on social media and joined the 6-Week Rapid Recovery Group Program.

At the time of starting the group she was seeking to gain weight, heal her chronic pain and renew her health. Within a few months she was able to heal her chronic pain, and throughout the past year continuing with a whole foods plant-based and oil-free lifestyle, gained 60lb returning to a place of embodied health and vitality.

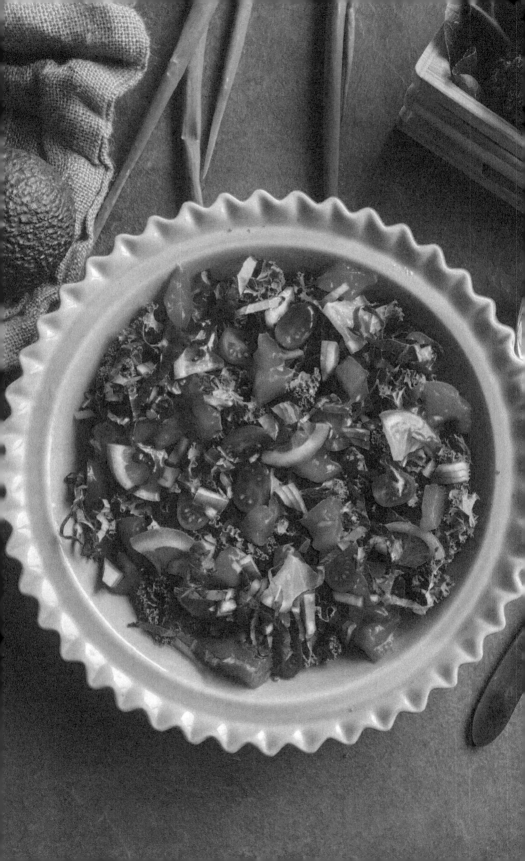

Mango Kale Salad

Ingredients:

1 bunch of kale	1 cup mango
1 avocado, peeled and pitted	1 pint cherry tomatoes
½ TB Braggs Liquid Aminos	¼ red onion
½ lime, juiced	

Method:

1. Coarsely chop the kale and place in a bowl with the avocado. Top with the lime juice and Braggs Liquid Aminos.

2. Massage the avocado, lime juice, and Braggs Liquid Aminos into the kale for a few minutes until the kale has wilted.

3. Chop the mango, cherry tomatoes, and red onion, and add these to the kale mixture. Stir to combine.

By Julie Teffeteller

In 2018, Julie was diagnosed with undifferentiated connective tissue disease. She suffered from various aches and pains, extreme digestive issues, and generalized anxiety. Following her diagnosis, she spent six months trying to heal through a Paleo/ Keto diet and a vast amount of very expensive supplements. While her digestive issues had improved, her pain had significantly increased.

In the summer of 2019, Julie switched to a vegan diet. She ate a lot of fruit, whole grains, and cooked vegetables, but she ate very little greens or healthy fats. She also frequently enjoyed vegan processed foods like rolled oats, rice, pasta, chips, and home baked treats. Her pain levels began to decrease and her digestion issues completely resolved, but she began experiencing significant nervous system issues including high levels of anxiety, tingles, and heart palpitations that woke her in the middle of the night. She was extremely fatigued. She could not work or keep up with her two young boys, and she was afraid to travel too far from home because of her symptoms.

In 2021, Julie enrolled in Dr. Goldner's 4 week one-on-one Rapid Recovery program. Upon completion, she continued the Rapid Recovery protocol on her own after for another4 weeks. After 6 weeks on protocol, her pain had completely disappeared, her energy levels were consistently high all day, and her anxiety had reduced by at least 75%. More importantly, she had the energy to keep up with her boys, and she returned to activities she used to love like going to the beach, visiting theme parks, and boating.

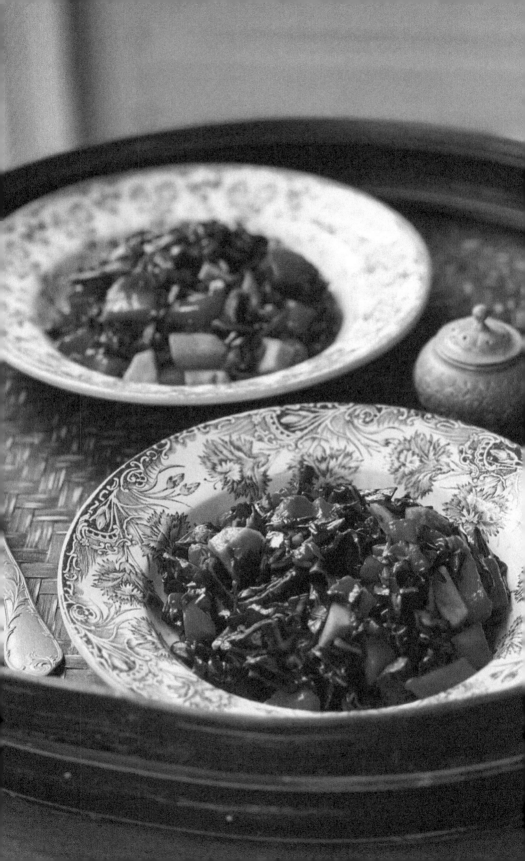

Red Cabbage Mango Salad

Ingredients:

7 oz red cabbage, finely chopped

7 oz fresh mango, in small pieces

2 oz apple, in small pieces

½ limes, juiced

Salt and pepper to taste

Method:

1. Mix all ingredients together and add salt and pepper to taste.

Recipe Note: It tastes even better when it marinates, so you can make it and take it with you to eat later.

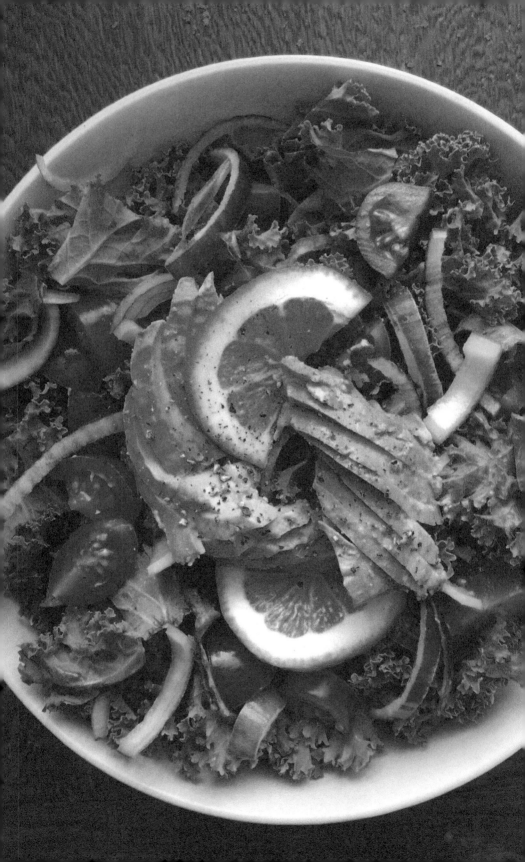

Refreshing Kale Salad

Ingredients:

2 cups kale or arugula

1 lemon, juiced

1 tsp salt

1/4 tsp black pepper

1 cup cherry tomatoes, cut into quarters or halves

1 red onion, thinly sliced

1 avocado, cubed or sliced

1 piece of seasonal fruit, cubed or sliced (my favorites are mango, apple, and pear)

Optional:

Red chili flakes for a spicy kick

Method:

1. Massage the greens with the lemon juice, salt, and pepper.

2. Top with remaining ingredients and a further squeeze of lemon juice.

By Nina Reyes Rosenberg

When I began Dr. Goldner's 6-Week Rapid Recovery Group, I was desperate. I had recently been diagnosed with systemic lupus erythematosus (SLE) and had rashes all over my face and head, arthritis, hair loss, fatigue, and brain fog. I was told there was no cure and would need to avoid sunlight for the rest of my life.

Within a month of doing Rapid Recovery, I was in the best shape of my life, I had no more pain, and my hair was growing back. At the end of the 6 weeks, my inflammation level was within normal range and the signs of lupus in my blood started to disappear. Within 9 months, my blood was completely normal with both DSDNA and ANA negative.

The habits and knowledge I developed in Rapid Recovery still serve me today. I'm almost 3 years lupus free according to my blood labs. I bask in the sun, eat a mostly whole foods / plant-based diet, and take care of my physical and mental health like I never did before. There is nothing I can't do, and I've learned how to optimize my immune system and prioritize my wellness to make everything else in my life flourish. Thanks to Dr. G, my lupus diagnosis went from being a living nightmare to the best thing that ever happened to me.

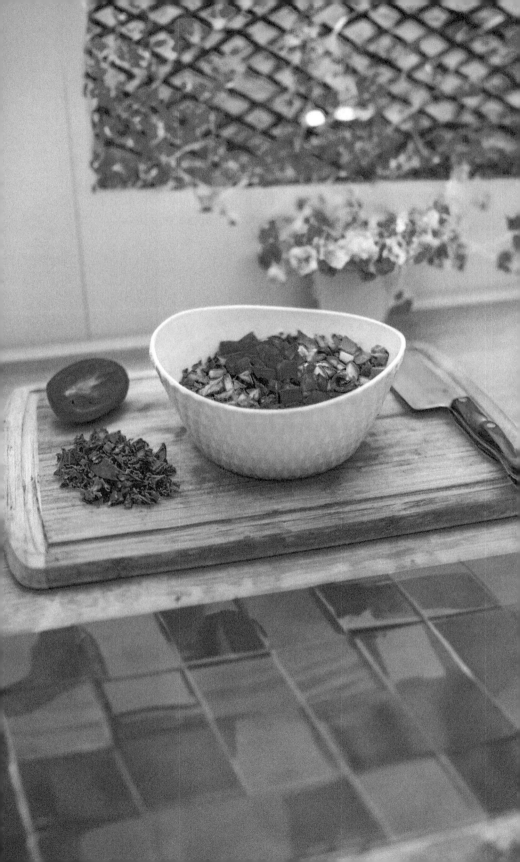

Chopped Salad

Ingredients:

3 oz spinach

1 oz kale

2 ½ oz red cabbage

4 ½ oz romaine lettuce

1 cucumber

1 Roma tomato

1 avocado (diced)

¼ cup or less pimento olives (in water)

1 tsp iodized salt

2 TB cold pressed flaxseed oil

2 TB balsamic vinegar (2g sugar or less per serving)

Method:

1. Place spinach, kale, red cabbage and lettuce in large wooden bowl and chop with mandolin knife. You can also use kitchen scissors or a food processor to chop to desired size (chopping makes it easier to eat especially large volumes).

2. Add cucumber, tomato, diced avocado, olives, salt, flaxseed oil and balsamic vinegar.

3. Mix and enjoy!

By Mary DiPalma

I joined the 6-Week Rapid Recovery Group after finding Dr. Goldner. I was diagnosed with RA in 2003, suffering with a lot of pain in my fingers, hands, wrists, arms, and shoulders. I also have osteoarthritis and am bone on bone in both my knees. I have lymphedema and am obese. I had to walk with a walker. I have heart failure and atrial fibrillation and my heart rate was always high. I was tired with low energy. I had anxiety and panic attacks along with agoraphobia and was homebound for over 4 years.

After finishing the 6-Week Rapid Recovery Group, I had much less pain in my knees and legs and NO more flare ups of pain in my fingers, hands, wrists, arms, and shoulders. I sleep much better now and have more energy. I am working out every day, walking better with less pain and even practicing walking with just a cane. Within a week after graduating from the group my heart rate normalized to the 60s and 70s from 110 to 115 before starting the Rapid Recovery Group.

My anxiety is so much better, and no more panic attacks. I am looking forward to getting out of my house for my daughter's wedding next and I will be dancing at her wedding with my husband.

I am truly blessed by finding Dr. Goldner and have enjoyed this salad every night.

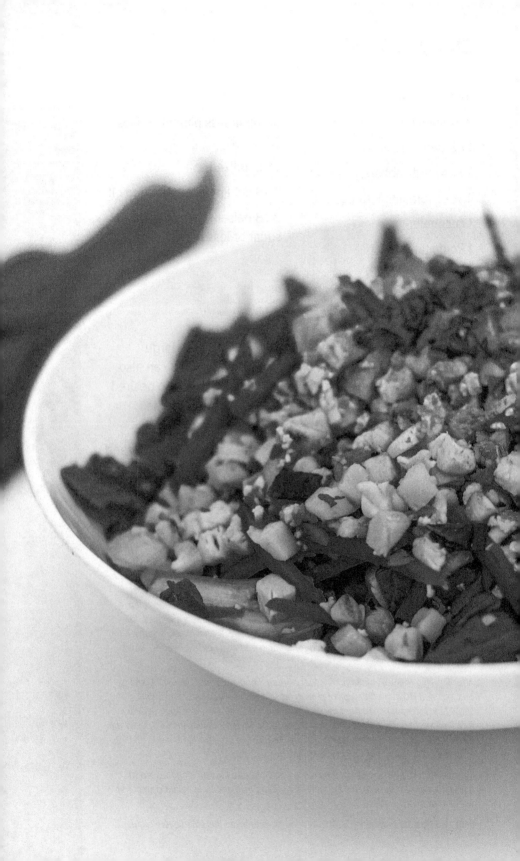

Crunchy Cauliflower and Bok Choy Medley

Ingredients:

5 oz cauliflower, chopped chunky or riced

5 oz bok choy, including the green tops, julienned

1 medium carrot, grated

½ medium onion, chopped

1-2 cloves garlic, minced

Handful cilantro, minced

3-4 TB lime juice

2 TB flaxseed oil

Salt (optional)

Pepper (optional)

Method:

1. Add all your prepped vegetables into one bowl. Add minced garlic and cilantro.

2. Squeeze limes and measure flaxseed oil and add to salad ingredients.

3. Toss to coat thoroughly. Salt and pepper to taste.

4. If you like nutritional yeast, make that your last add. You can toss in or sprinkle on top.

Recipe note: After dressing is tossed in, top with nutritional yeast

2-4 oz Purple Cabbage, finely shredded, for more color and nutrients!

By Joan Cothern

It's amazing how your body thanks you when you nourish it and how quickly it can happen! Who would have ever guessed that six weeks of the Rapid Recovery Group would cut my thyroid antibodies in half, lower my blood pressure to 100/70 and cut my inflammation marker (CRP) in half??!!!

None of these markers have moved in many years and six weeks made it happen. In addition my muscle and joint pain completely disappeared, making an hour-long walk possible and a pleasure. YAYYY for me!

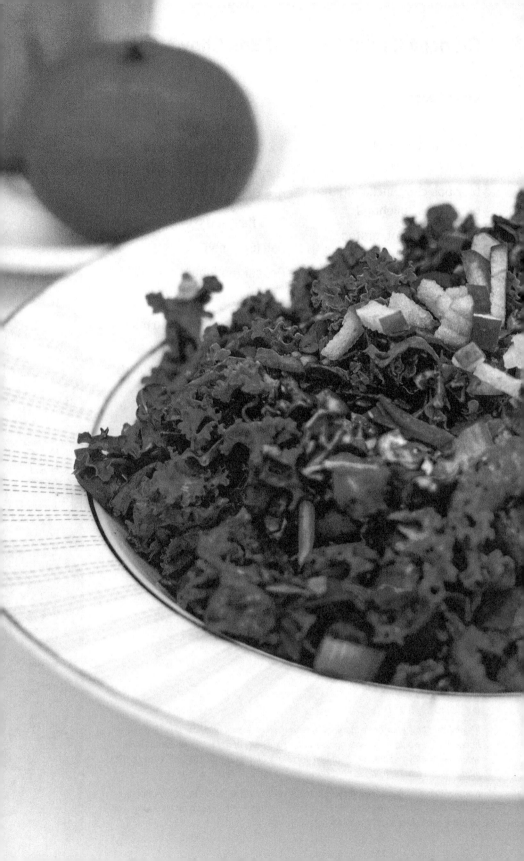

Citrusy Kale Ribbon Salad

Ingredients:

4-6 cups kale, chiffonade (in ribbon like strips)

2-3 cups purple cabbage, cut in super fine shreds

2 scallions, chopped

Orange rind from ½ orange, cut rind or peel in very thin strips, remove white pith.

¼ cup mint, chopped

¼ cup cilantro, chopped

1 apple, peeled and cut in small cubes (optional)

Dressing:

6 TB flax oil

4 TB rice wine vinegar

2 tsp tamari

1 garlic clove, minced

Dash of cayenne

Salt and pepper, to taste.

Recipe note: You can zest the other half of the orange and add it to the dressing if you like! It's yummy especially if you are adding the apples.

Method:

1. Place kale and cabbage in a bowl. Whisk all dressing ingredients together until emulsified a bit. Add to greens. Massage in with hands to tenderize the kale and cabbage.

2. Add the herbs and strips of orange peel along with the scallions and apple. Toss again. Enjoy!

By Joan Cothern

It's amazing how your body thanks you when you nourish it and how quickly it can happen! Who would have ever guessed that six weeks of the Rapid Recovery Group would cut my thyroid antibodies in half, lower my blood pressure to 100/70 and cut my inflammation marker (CRP) in half??!!!

None of these markers have moved in many years and six weeks made it happen. In addition my muscle and joint pain completely disappeared, making an hour-long walk possible and a pleasure. YAYYY for me!

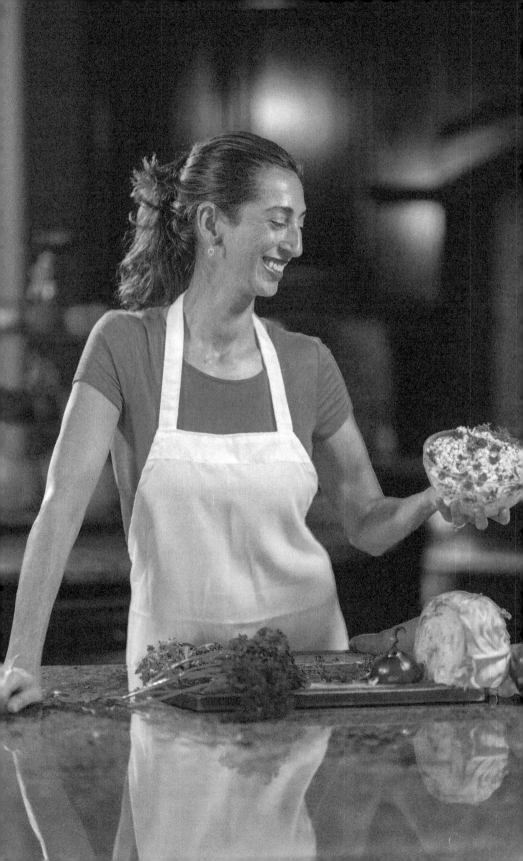

NUTRIENT-DENSE
MEALS

Recipes for when you want
health-giving meals that are fun and
hearty

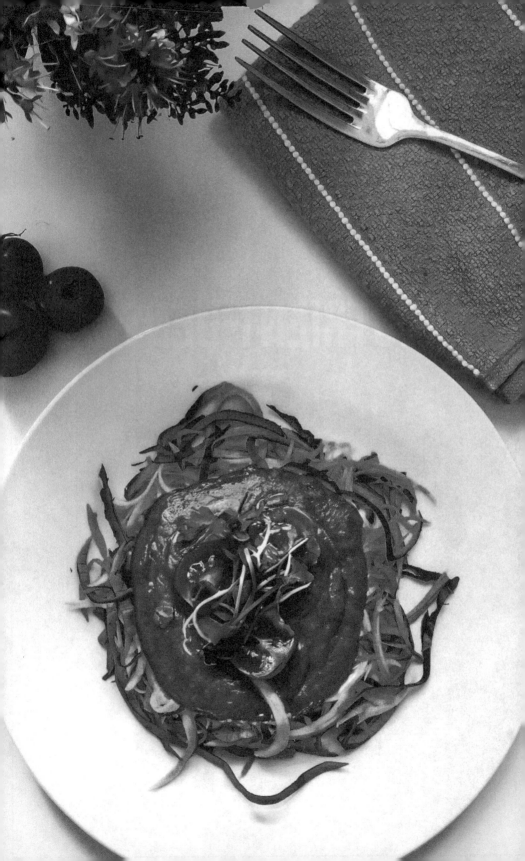

Dr. G's Zucchini Noodles with Marinara

Ingredients:

5 zucchinis (or yellow squash)

Sauce:

2 ½ cup chopped Roma tomatoes

2 TB Braggs Liquid Aminos

⅓ cup lemon juice

2 TB diced onions

2 TB garlic

0.25 oz fresh basil

Salt and pepper to taste

1-2 TB cold pressed flaxseed oil (optional)

Method:

1. Spiralize the zucchini into noodles. You can also use a mandolin or regular peeler to make long fettuccine-like ribbons.
2. Place sauce ingredients in a high-speed blender.
3. Blend until smooth but don't let it heat up.
4. Pour over the zucchini noodles and toss.

By Brooke Goldner, M.D.

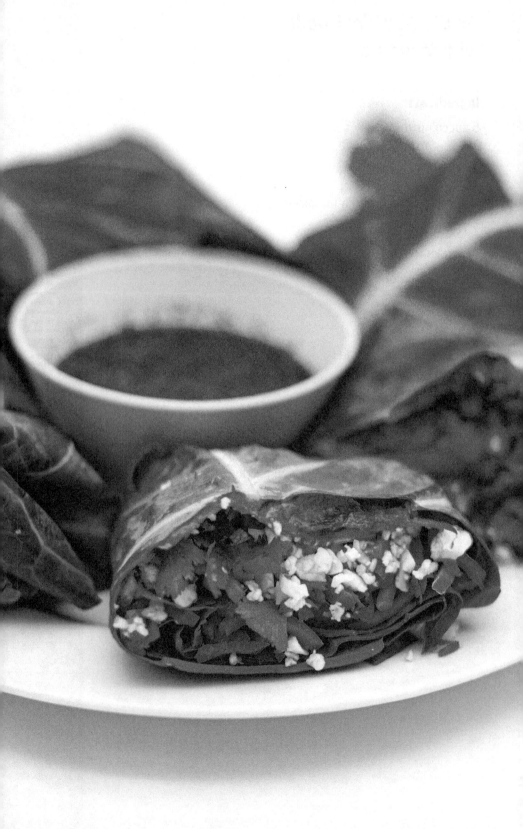

Collard Spring Rolls with Flax Dipping Sauce

Ingredients:

2 collard leaves

½ large avocado

½ cup of riced cauliflower

⅓ cup of radishes, thinly sliced

⅓ cup of carrots, cut into thin strips

⅓ cup of cucumbers, cut into thin strips

2 TB of cilantro leaves

Dipping Sauce Ingredients:

2 tsp freshly ground flaxseeds

1 TB rice wine vinegar

1 TB Braggs Liquid Aminos

1 tsp lime juice

½ tsp grated ginger

¼ tsp sugar-free hot sauce or red pepper flakes to taste

1 tsp avocado

Method:

1. Use collard leaves that are room temperature or rinse under warm water and pat dry. Lay the leaf flat with the stem side up and use a small knife or a peeler to shave back the thick part of the stem that runs up the middle of the leaf.

2. Mash the avocado and spread it in the middle of the leaf. Then add the cauliflower rice, radishes, carrots, cucumbers, and cilantro.

3. Roll the leaf like a burrito, cut in half, and serve with the dipping sauce.

Method for the Dipping Sauce

1. Blend all dipping sauce ingredients in a blender until all ingredients are well combined. Alternatively, mix or whisk by hand.

2. Serve with collard wrap.

By Lexi W.

I am so grateful to have found Dr. G. I was at a low point in my 30-plus year battle with Lupus/Sjogren's. After doing 1:1 Rapid Recovery with Dr. G, not only did I improve all areas of inflammation, and there were many, but I got off my steroids for the first time in 30 years! I also stopped taking daily naps and had high energy levels for the first time since my twenties. Dr. G taught me that the body is designed to heal itself, given the proper nutrients. I saw that fact with my very own eyes after needing stitches while doing Rapid Recovery; my skin healed in the standard 10-day time period as opposed to the several months it has required in the past. This recipe is my take on a spring roll and I hope you enjoy it!

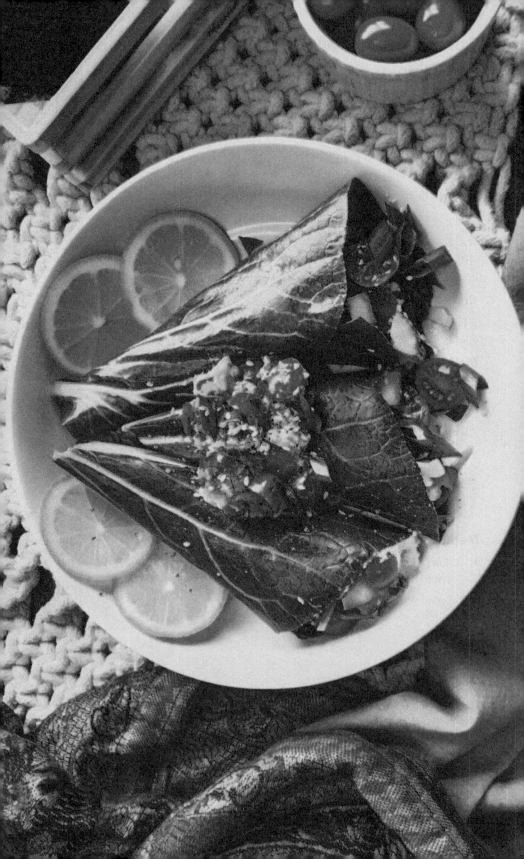

Collard Wraps

Ingredients:

2 large collard leaves

1 large avocado, pitted and sliced

1 tsp Dijon mustard

1 TB lemon juice

½ cup cherry tomatoes, chopped

½ cup cucumber, chopped

½ cup shredded carrots

¼ cup red bell pepper

½ cup sprouts

Salt and pepper to taste

Method:

1. Wash and dry the collard leaves, and then use a small paring knife to cut out the base of the stem.

2. In a bowl, mash the avocado with the mustard, lemon juice, and salt and pepper. Spread half of this mixture on each of the collard leaves.

3. Reuse that same bowl to combine the remaining ingredients. Mix well. Distribute evenly between the collard leaves.

4. Roll each collard wrap up like a burrito by first folding up the bottom edge (lengthwise), then folding in the sides, and then rolling up to the top edge.

Recipe note: For more flavor dip into Braggs Liquid Aminos, fresh salsa, or more mustard.

By Julie Teffeteller

In 2018, Julie was diagnosed with undifferentiated connective tissue disease. She suffered from various aches and pains, extreme digestive issues, and generalized anxiety. Following her diagnosis, she spent six months trying to heal through a Paleo/ Keto diet and a vast amount of very expensive supplements. While her digestive issues had improved, her pain had significantly increased.

In the summer of 2019, Julie switched to a vegan diet. She ate a lot of fruit, whole grains, and cooked vegetables, but she ate very little greens or healthy fats. She also frequently enjoyed vegan processed foods like rolled oats, rice, pasta, chips, and home baked treats. Her pain levels began to decrease and her digestion issues completely resolved, but she began experiencing significant nervous system issues including high levels of anxiety, tingles, and heart palpitations that woke her in the middle of the night. She was extremely fatigued. She could not work or keep up with her two young boys, and she was afraid to travel too far from home because of her symptoms.

In 2021, Julie enrolled in Dr. Goldner's 4 week one-on-one Rapid Recovery program. Upon completion, she continued the Rapid Recovery protocol on her own after for another4 weeks. After 6 weeks on protocol, her pain had completely disappeared, her energy levels were consistently high all day, and her anxiety had reduced by at least 75%. More importantly, she had the energy to keep up with her boys, and she returned to activities she used to love like going to the beach, visiting theme parks, and boating.

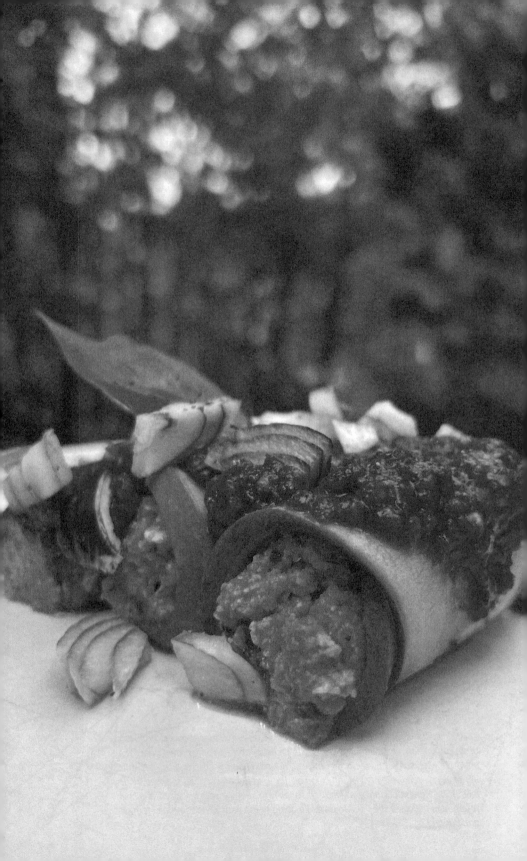

Zucchini Cannelloni

Ingredients:

2 large zucchinis

1 red onion

1 avocado

½ head of cauliflower

2 garlic cloves

3 TB nutritional yeast

2 TB flaxseed oil

¼ cup fresh basil

2 sprigs chopped fresh rosemary

1 sprig fresh thyme

4 TB Braggs Liquid Aminos

½ cup water

Salt and pepper to taste

¾ cup Roma tomatoes

2 cups cherry tomatoes

3 TB balsamic vinegar (optional)

Instructions:

1. Using a vegetable slicer, or mandolin cut the zucchini very finely into long strips that can bend.

2. In a small bowl mix the flaxseed oil, water, Braggs Liquid Aminos, ½ tsp salt, fresh rosemary and coat the zucchini. Set aside.

3. Using a food processor, add the cauliflower and process, not long just a few times.

4. Then add ½ avocado, nutritional yeast, nearly all the basil, thyme, 1 clove garlic and salt and pepper. Process until combined.

5. With the zucchini strips place the cauliflower mixture into the middle and roll up. Do that with the rest of the zucchini strips.

6. Empty the food processor and add all of the tomatoes and remainder garlic, and remainder basil leaves and 2 TB balsamic vinegar. Blend until combined well.

7. Spoon tomato mixture on top of zucchini. Top with red onion and avocado with salt and pepper to taste.

By Robyn Lawley

Barely 2 months after my daughter was born, I had multiple strokes caused by a blood clotting disorder called APS and was diagnosed with lupus. The strokes caused post-stroke epilepsy. After several bad seizures and zero hope from the doctors, I decided to give Dr. Goldner a call.

Dr. Goldner's protocol helped put my very aggressive lupus into remission, and turn my very scary bloody clotting disorder APS from positive to negative on my blood reports.

I completed Dr. Goldner's Rapid Recovery program in March 2019. November 2019, my rheumatologist called to advise me my diet had been contributing to my health and I no longer had to take medication for my lupus and APS.

I owe my life to Dr. Goldner! She helped me have the courage to take care of my own body and destiny. Thank you once again for getting rid of my lupus! Do her program BEFORE you suffer the damage!

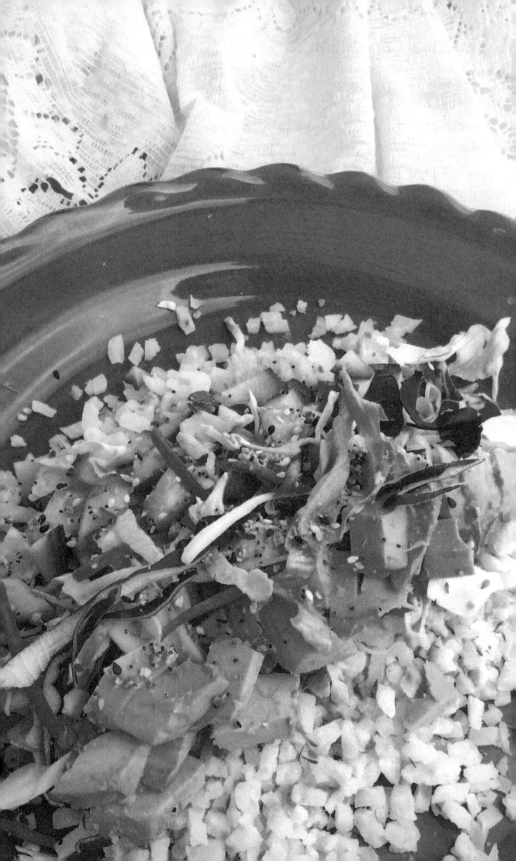

Sushi Rice

Ingredients:

12 oz cauliflower

2 sheets dried nori

⅓ cup cabbage, chopped

1 bell pepper, chopped

⅓ cup cucumber, chopped

⅓ cup shredded carrots

1 avocado, diced

1 TB Braggs Liquid Aminos

Method:

1. Add the cauliflower and the dried nori to a food processor or a blender and pulse until the cauliflower is chopped into rice sized pieces.

2. Place the cauliflower rice in a bowl.

3. Top with remaining chopped vegetables, season with the Braggs Liquid Aminos, and stir.

By Julie Teffeteller

In 2018, Julie was diagnosed with undifferentiated connective tissue disease. She suffered from various aches and pains, extreme digestive issues, and generalized anxiety. Following her diagnosis, she spent six months trying to heal through a Paleo/ Keto diet and a vast amount of very expensive supplements. While her digestive issues had improved, her pain had significantly increased.

In the summer of 2019, Julie switched to a vegan diet. She ate a lot of fruit, whole grains, and cooked vegetables, but she ate very little greens or healthy fats. She also frequently enjoyed vegan processed foods like rolled oats, rice, pasta, chips, and home baked treats. Her pain levels began to decrease and her digestion issues completely resolved, but she began experiencing significant nervous system issues including high levels of anxiety, tingles, and heart palpitations that woke her in the middle of the night. She was extremely fatigued. She could not work or keep up with her two young boys, and she was afraid to travel too far from home because of her symptoms.

In 2021, Julie enrolled in Dr. Goldner's 4 week one-on-one Rapid Recovery program. Upon completion, she continued the Rapid Recovery protocol on her own after for another4 weeks. After 6 weeks on protocol, her pain had completely disappeared, her energy levels were consistently high all day, and her anxiety had reduced by at least 75%. More importantly, she had the energy to keep up with her boys, and she returned to activities she used to love like going to the beach, visiting theme parks, and boating.

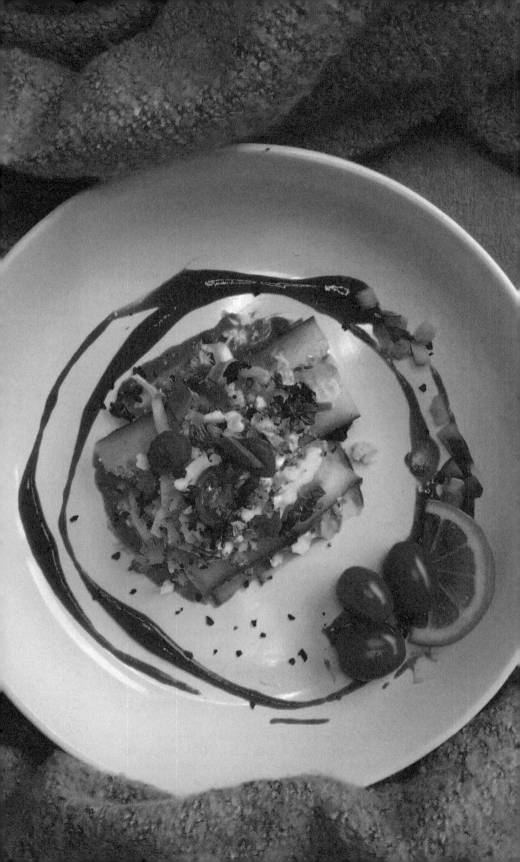

Dr. G's Cruciferous Lasagna

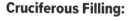

Ingredients:

Cruciferous Filling:

1 cup broccoli

1 cup cauliflower

1 TB Braggs Aminos

Tomato Filling:

1 cup cherry tomatoes

1 handful fresh basil

1 clove garlic

Salt and pepper to taste

Guacamole Filling:

2 avocados

½ tsp salt

1 ½ TB lemon juice

1 clove minced garlic

Noodles:

1 medium zucchini

Method:

1. Slice zucchini into thin lengthwise slices with a mandolin or sharp knife. These will be your lasagna noodles.

2. Prepare cruciferous filling: pulse broccoli and cauliflower in a food processor or chop by hand. Mix in Braggs Liquid Aminos and put aside.

3. Prepare tomato filling: add tomatoes, basil, and garlic to the food processor and mix until well combined. Mix in salt and pepper to taste.

4. Prepare guacamole filling: smash avocados with a fork or pulse in a food processor. Add lemon juice, garlic and salt and mix well.

5. Assemble lasagna: put 2 slices of your lasagna "noodles" on your plate. Add a layer of guacamole. Add a layer of tomato filling. Add a layer of your cruciferous veggies. Then put another 2 pieces of zucchini noodles down. Repeat the process until your tower of lasagna is complete!

6. Serve immediately or store in the refrigerator.

By Brooke Goldner, M.D.

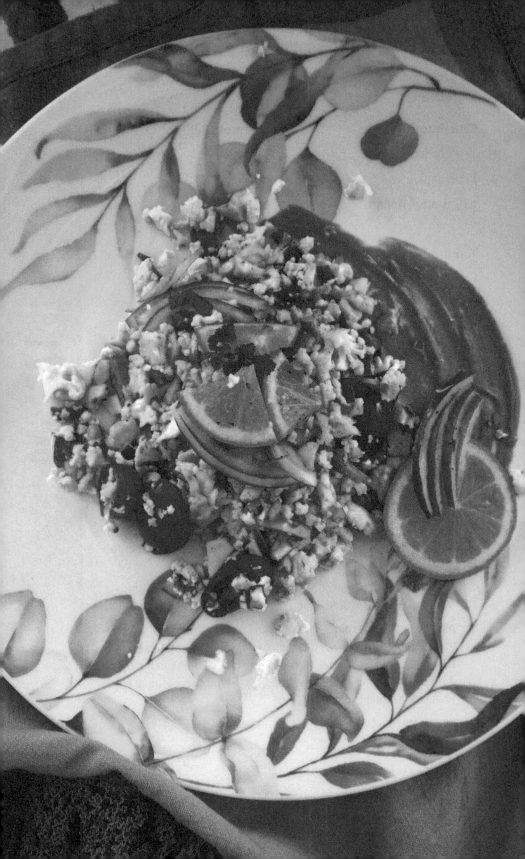

Cauliflower Risotto

Ingredients:

1 ½ cups cauliflower florets (or mix of cauliflower and broccoli)

1 avocado

3-4 cherry tomatoes or ½ cup of sweet potato

1 tsp cumin

Pinch of salt and pepper

2 TB lemon juice

2 TB of basil and/or parsley

1 tsp of tamari (optional)

Method:

1. Place cauliflower in a food processor and process into a fine rice consistency.

2. Transfer cauliflower to a bowl, and add the remaining ingredients.

3. Mix until still risotto consistency, not a paste

By Tina Trtnik

My name is Tina and I was into sports all my life, until a few years ago when inflammation in one knee started to appear for the first time. It got better after steroid injections for a couple of years. But the next time it appeared in both knees, and aspiration and steroids did not help any more. I was pretty much home, resting my legs and missed sports like crazy.

Now that I think back, I can see I had all the signs of autoimmune disease from my teenage years. I had migraines a lot, and they grew more frequent as I aged. I was constipated a lot and nothing helped. I had anxiety and brittle hair. There were numerous signs that my body was not happy and needed help.

I joined Dr. Goldner's 6 Week Rapid Recovery group in May, right before my birthday. I didn't care about anything else, I just wanted my life back. I needed to change everything, not only food, but my outlook on life. I had to learn how to overcome my emotional blockages and learn to think differently, because the life I was living before had driven me to disease.

My knees were pain-free after the group ended, and I kept working on my emotions and food even after I healed. Today I am great. My health has never been better.

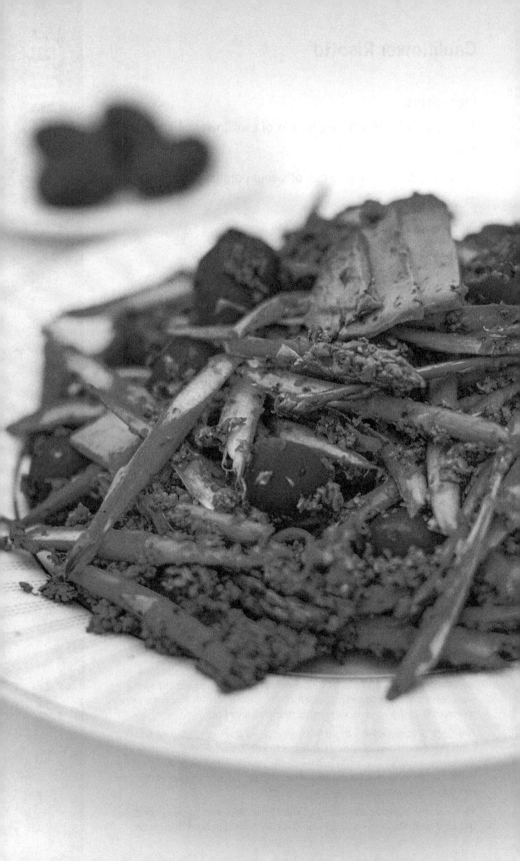

Asparagus Pesto Salad

Salad Ingredients:

2 cups sliced asparagus

1 cup cherry tomatoes

1 avocado, finely sliced

Pesto Ingredients:

½ cup basil

1 cup broccoli

3 TB nutritional yeast

Salt and pepper to taste

5 TB of cold pressed flaxseed oil

Cayenne and chili powder (optional)

Method:

1. Combine pesto ingredients in a food processor and pulse to desired consistency.

2. Combine salad ingredients with the pesto and serve.

By Tina Trtnik

My name is Tina and I was into sports all my life, until a few years ago when inflammation in one knee started to appear for the first time. It got better after steroid injections for a couple of years. But the next time it appeared in both knees, and aspiration and steroids did not help any more. I was pretty much home, resting my legs and missed sports like crazy.

Now that I think back, I can see I had all the signs of autoimmune disease from my teenage years. I had migraines a lot, and they grew more frequent as I aged. I was constipated a lot and nothing helped. I had anxiety and brittle hair. There were numerous signs that my body was not happy and needed help.

I joined Dr. Goldner's 6 Week Rapid Recovery group in May, right before my birthday. I didn't care about anything else, I just wanted my life back. I needed to change everything, not only food, but my outlook on life. I had to learn how to overcome my emotional blockages and learn to think differently, because the life I was living before had driven me to disease.

My knees were pain-free after the group ended, and I kept working on my emotions and food even after I healed. Today I am great. My health has never been better.

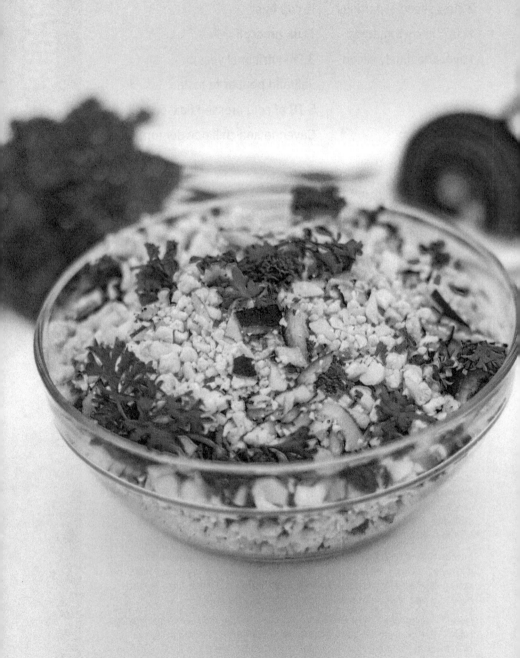

Cauliflower Slaw

Ingredients:

5 cups cauliflower

1 ½ cups purple onion

½ cup parsley

1 tsp pepper

Method:

1. Chop the first three ingredients and combine in a bowl.

2. Top with pepper and mix well.

3. Serve with Dr. G's Raw Avocado Caesar Salad Dressing (page 111).

By Annette Rio Hennesey

I joined Rapid Recovery because I was having some strange shocks throughout my body that none of my doctors could diagnose.

The shocks went away in the first 6 weeks of starting the Rapid Recovery Group! However, the most drastic improvements came later.

Many years ago, I was a marathoner. A drunk driver broke both of my legs. After seven surgeries and countless hours of physical therapy, my doctors told me that my pain wasn't going to get any better and that my distance running was over.

But, after a year of hyper-nourishing, I realized that it had been a long time since my legs had really hurt. I decided to see just how much activity they could handle.

Since then, I have been doing 50-miles per week and my legs feel GREAT! I just registered for my first marathon since I was injured. I also now have a negative ANA!

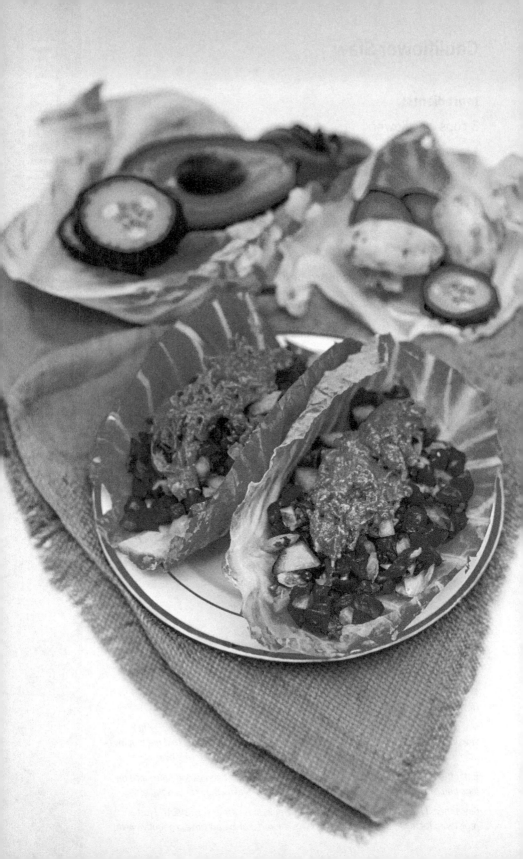

Dr. G's Raw Tasty Tacos

Ingredients:

Green cabbage (or romaine lettuce)

2 cups riced cauliflower

2 TB Braggs Liquid Aminos

2 mushrooms, diced

1 medium cucumber, diced

Gourmet Guacamole (page 115)
Pico de Gallo (page 97)

Instructions:

1. Add Braggs Liquid Aminos, riced cauliflower and diced mushrooms to a bowl.

2. Mix until fully coated, and put aside.

3. Take a cabbage or romaine lettuce leaf and place it on a plate.

4. Add 2-3 TB of cauliflower and cucumber to the leaf (depending on the size of the leaf and what it can hold).

5. Top with cucumbers and any other veggies you like.

6. Top with pico de gallo and guacamole to taste

7. Wrap the sides of the leaf closed, pick it up and eat it!

Recipe note: You can use store-bought pre-cut riced cauliflower, or chop it in a food processor, or use a sharp knife to cut to size. Add any extra veggies you like for more flavor.

By Brooke Goldner, M.D.

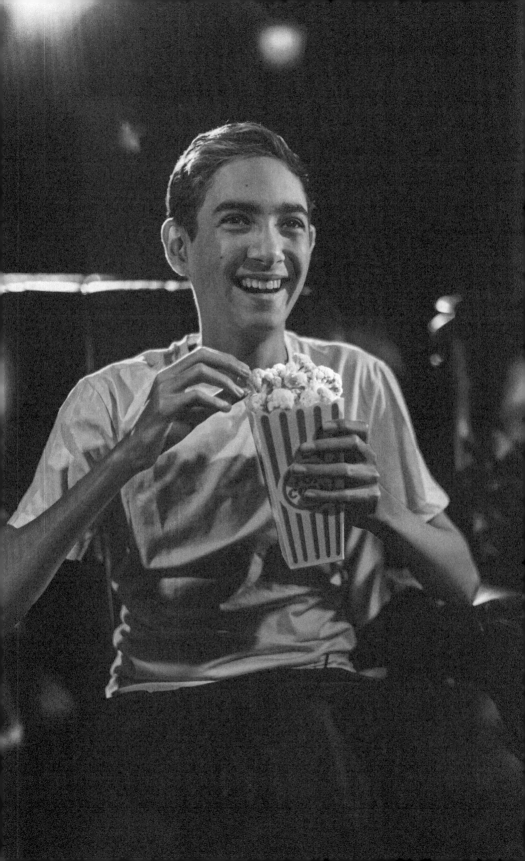

SATISFYING
SNACKS

These are some of my favorite healthy snacks that I keep around for when I crave something savory and exciting or if I am serving up snacks for company.

— Brooke Goldner, M.D.

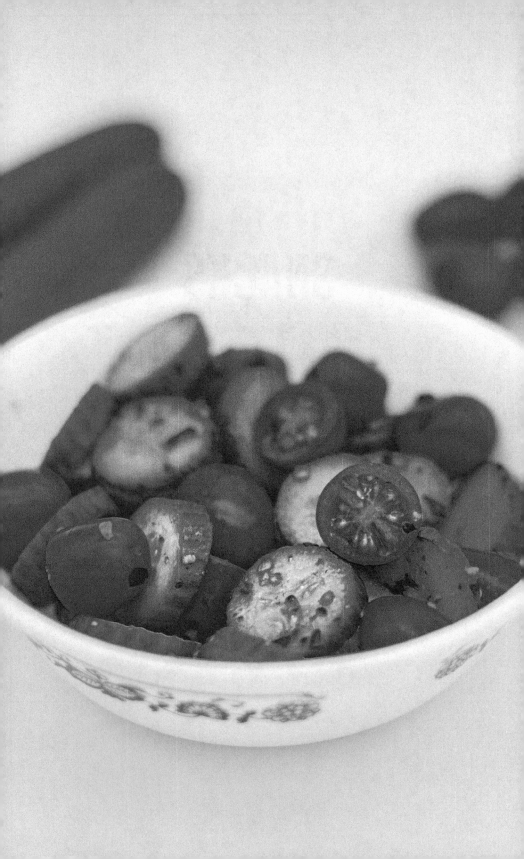

Ginger Cucumber Salad

Ingredients:

2 Japanese cucumbers

10 cherry tomatoes

Pinch of salt and pepper

3 TB apple vinegar

1 medium chili finely chopped or 1 tsp of chili flakes

2 garlic cloves (grated)

Nub of ginger (grated)

Method:

1. Slice the cucumbers and remove seeds. Slice diagonally and place in a bowl.

2. Add salt and sit for 10 minutes.

3. Gently squeeze any water from the cucumber and add tomatoes.

4. Mix all the remaining dressing ingredients in a small bowl.

5. Pour dressing over the salad and toss to combine.

By Tina Trtnik

My name is Tina and I was into sports all my life, until a few years ago when inflammation in one knee started to appear for the first time. It got better after steroid injections for a couple of years. But the next time it appeared in both knees, and aspiration and steroids did not help any more. I was pretty much home, resting my legs and missed sports like crazy.

Now that I think back, I can see I had all the signs of autoimmune disease from my teenage years. I had migraines a lot, and they grew more frequent as I aged. I was constipated a lot and nothing helped. I had anxiety and brittle hair. There were numerous signs that my body was not happy and needed help.

I joined Dr. Goldner's 6 Week Rapid Recovery group in May, right before my birthday. I didn't care about anything else, I just wanted my life back. I needed to change everything, not only food, but my outlook on life. I had to learn how to overcome my emotional blockages and learn to think differently, because the life I was living before had driven me to disease.

My knees were pain-free after the group ended, and I kept working on my emotions and food even after I healed. Today I am great. My health has never been better.

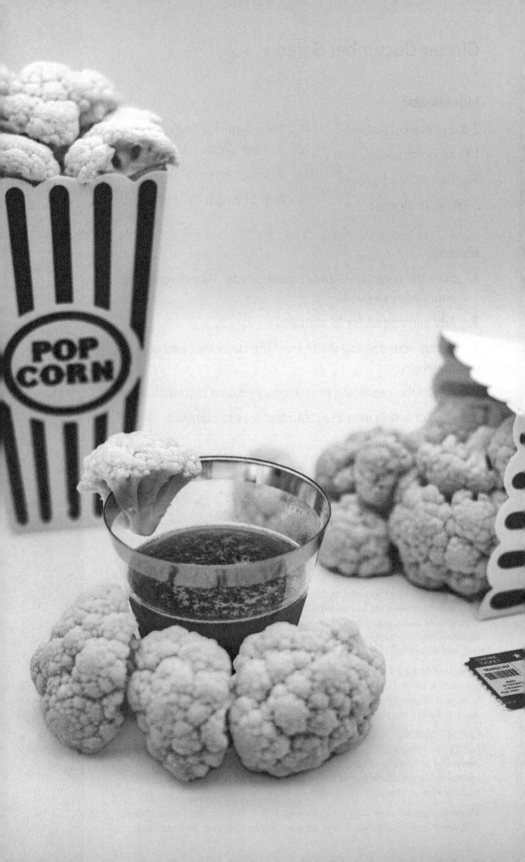

Buttered Popcorn Dip

Ingredients:

1 TB nutritional yeast

3 TB flaxseed oil

1 tsp turmeric

¼-1 tsp salt

½ tsp cinnamon (optional)

Dash of a sugar free hot sauce (optional)

1 small head of cauliflower cut into bite size pieces

Method:

1. Add the first 6 ingredients to a small bowl and whisk together.

2. For a fun finger food, just dip pieces of cauliflower into the bowl and eat.

3. Alternatively, you can toss the cauliflower with the rest of the ingredients and serve as a snack that you eat with a fork.

By Anonymous

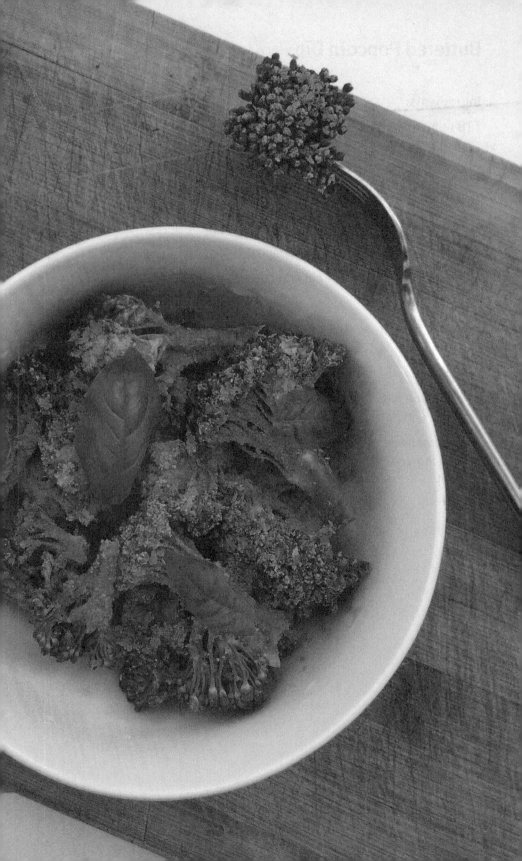

Cheezy Broccoli Snack

Ingredients:

1 cup broccoli

1 TB nutritional yeast

Garlic salt to taste

Method:

1. Rinse broccoli to help the other ingredients stick.

2. Sprinkle the broccoli with the remaining ingredients and mix well.

By Ashley Daniels Lawther

I have psoriatic arthritis. I've had joint pain since I was 8 years old. My disease started getting progressively worse, I was having to double up on my medication and even that was not cutting the pain. Stomach pain attacks would last for about an hour, they were very debilitating, I would sometimes almost pass out from the pain. I couldn't run, I was having difficulty walking, and I was having trouble cooking and doing the dishes. So, I knew I needed to do something different and so I signed up with Dr. Goldner.

Within 30 days my joint pain was significantly better. By the end of the Rapid Recovery program I had no more joint pain. I can run no problem, I have no problem walking. My stomach pain also completely went away. I lost about 10 pounds. My nails are very long and I feel really good. It feels so nice not to just like wake up in the morning and your body feels so good. Like you can move, you can move freely, nothing hurts. I'm so happy I did this and I would definitely recommend this for you all as well.

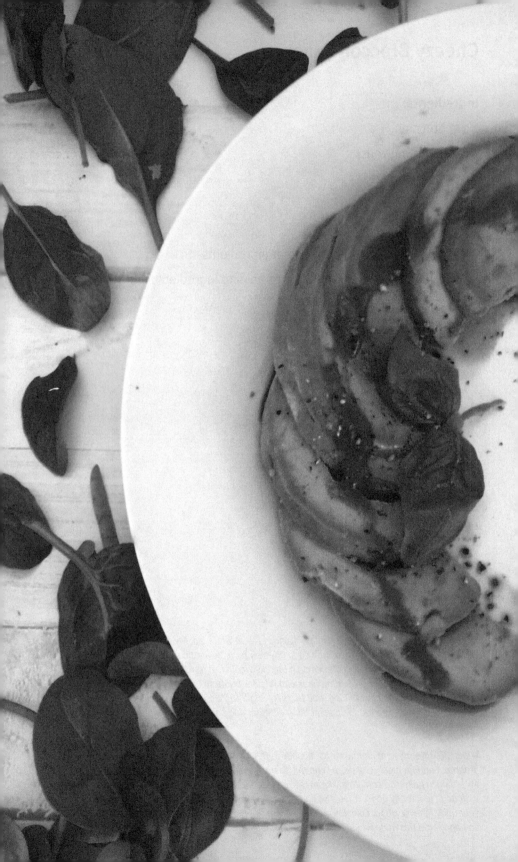

Dr. G's Avocado Snack

Ingredients:

1 avocado

Braggs Liquid Aminos, to taste

Nutritional yeast, to taste

Few dots of sugar free hot sauce

Method:

1. Pit, peel, and slice the avocado.
2. Season to taste with a few drops of Braggs Liquid Aminos, a sprinkle of nutritional yeast, and a few dots of sugar free hot sauce.

By Brooke Goldner, M.D.

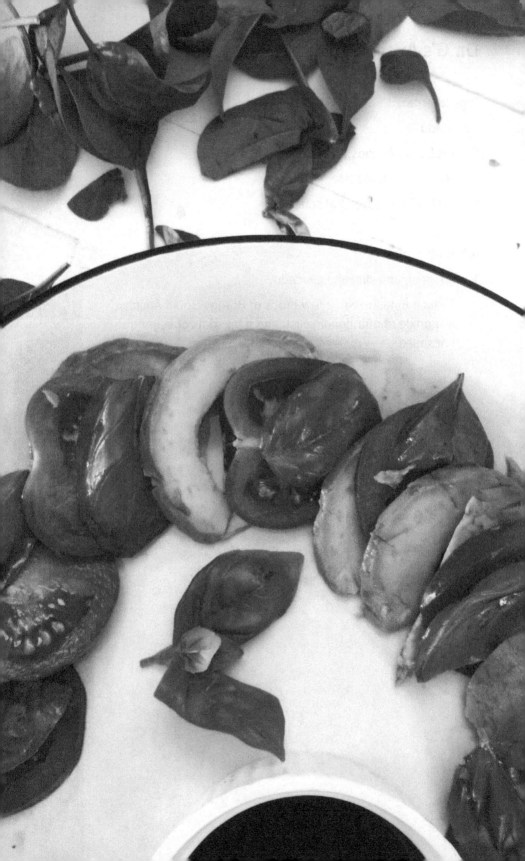

Vegan Caprese

Ingredients:

2 tomatoes, sliced

½ bunch basil, leaves only

1 avocado, diced

Balsamic vinegar for drizzling

Method:

1. Stack one slice of tomato, one basil leaf, and one avocado chunk.
2. Repeat with remaining ingredients.
3. Drizzle with balsamic vinegar.

By Allie Warren

I was first diagnosed with discoid lupus and was later diagnosed with systemic lupus while pregnant with my first child, which added some stress during my pregnancy.

After having my daughter, I came across Dr. Goldner. I bought her books and ended up joining the 6-Week Rapid Recovery Group. I wanted to make sure I was doing everything correctly so that my body could heal. I wanted to be healthy enough to see my daughter grow up.

Since the 6-Week Rapid Recovery Group, I have been feeling great! I continue to drink a full pitcher of smoothie every day and had another successful pregnancy!

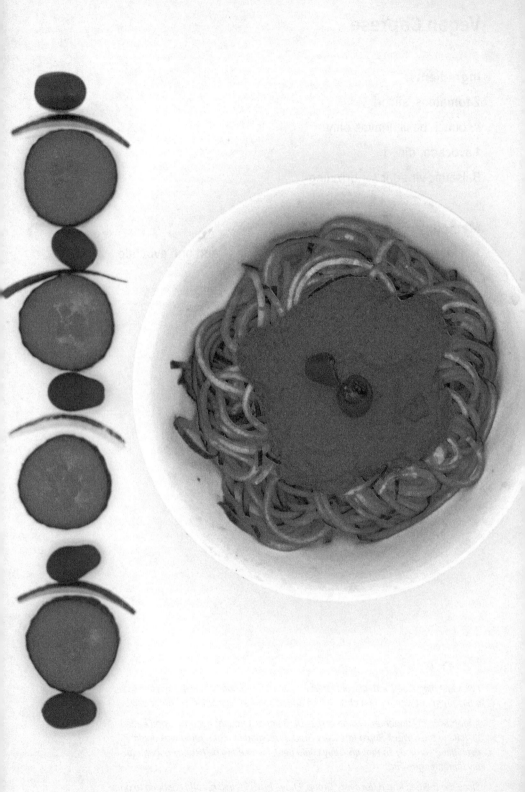

Cucumber Noodles with Tomato Sauce

Ingredients:

1 large cucumber

1 pint cherry tomatoes

3 garlic cloves

¼ red onion

1 TB flax oil

¼ cup nutritional yeast

Salt to taste

Method:

1. Spiralize the cucumber.
2. Place all other ingredients in a high speed blender in the order listed.
3. Blend until smooth, adding water as needed to thin.
4. Pour sauce over the spiralized cucumber and enjoy.

By Hilda Moleski

I struggled with deep fatigue and being overweight. I lost 13 pounds during the 6-Week Rapid Recovery Group and felt remarkably energetic by the end of the six weeks!

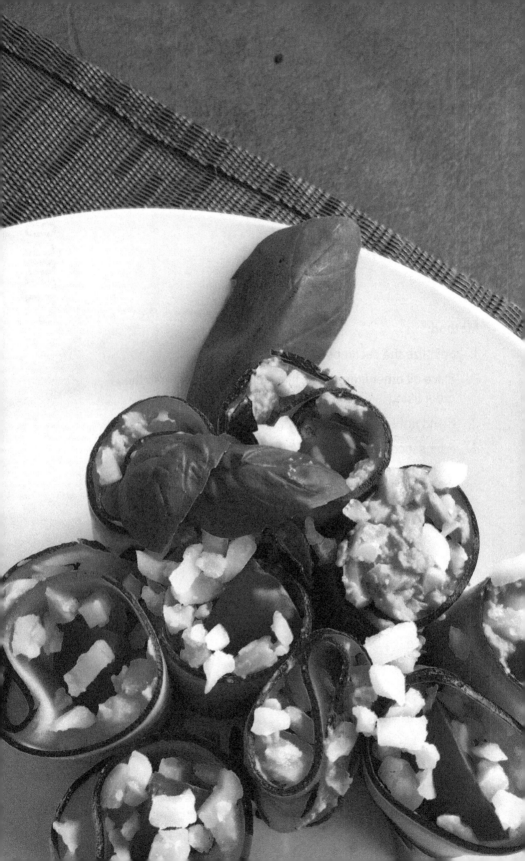

Zucchini Rolls

Ingredients:

1 cup zucchini, sliced with knife or mandolin

1 cup mixed cauliflower, broccoli, red cabbage, scallion

1 cup guacamole

½ cup cherry tomatoes, halved

Braggs Liquid Aminos

Oregano for garnish

Method:

1. Spread guacamole on a zucchini slice and season with Braggs Liquid Aminos.

2. Add a small scoop of the chopped mixture on top of the guacamole. Then, in the middle, add part of a tomato.

3. Roll the zucchini and add oregano on top.

By Anonymous

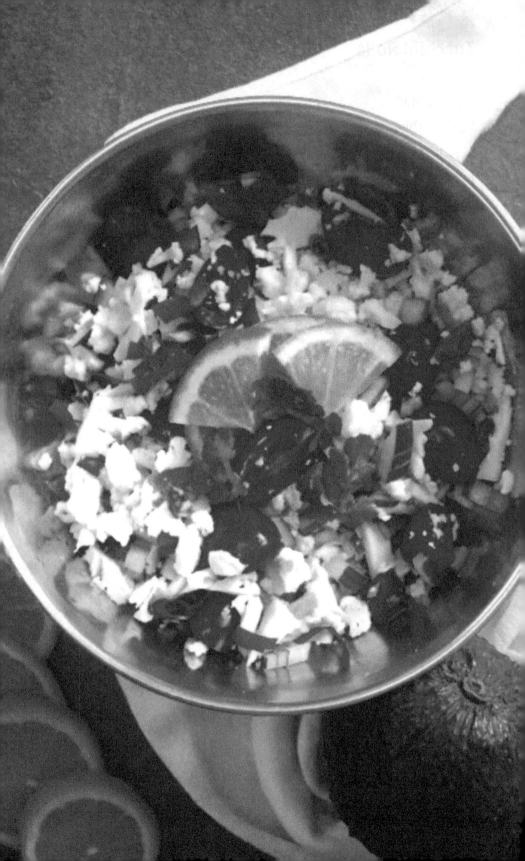

Cauliflower Ceviche

Ingredients:

1 head cauliflower

4 lemons

4 tomatoes

1 red onion

1 bunch of cilantro

Salt to taste

Method:

1. Place cauliflower in a food processor and process into a fine consistency.

2. Transfer cauliflower to a bowl, add the juice of 2 lemons and add salt to taste. Let it marinate.

3. Meanwhile, dice tomatoes, onion, and cilantro. Add to the marinated cauliflower.

4. Squeeze the other two lemons over top and mix. Let it sit for an hour before serving.

By Laura Rivero

I remember when I heard about Dr. Brooke Goldner through another website. I read/ heard her story and started looking for more information. I finally contacted her. We scheduled a consultation phone call where I explained to her what I was going through. At the time, I had been struggling with a lot of pain. I had been diagnosed with RA, Lyme, anemia and my inflammation markers were off the charts high! Her enthusiasm is so real and nurturing that I decided to do her 6-Week Rapid Recovery Program.

The 6-Week Rapid Recovery Program was very eye opening. It helped me realize how and why I got to where I was. I had been neglecting myself for years! I love my family, but it's so true that to take care of others, you need to care for yourself first. The program was what I needed to get a boost into my recovery. I felt better, lost weight, which is an awesome side effect!

After her program, I continued eating a plant-based diet. I am now living pain free. I want to thank you Dr. G for everything you did for me and for everything you continue to do. God bless you.

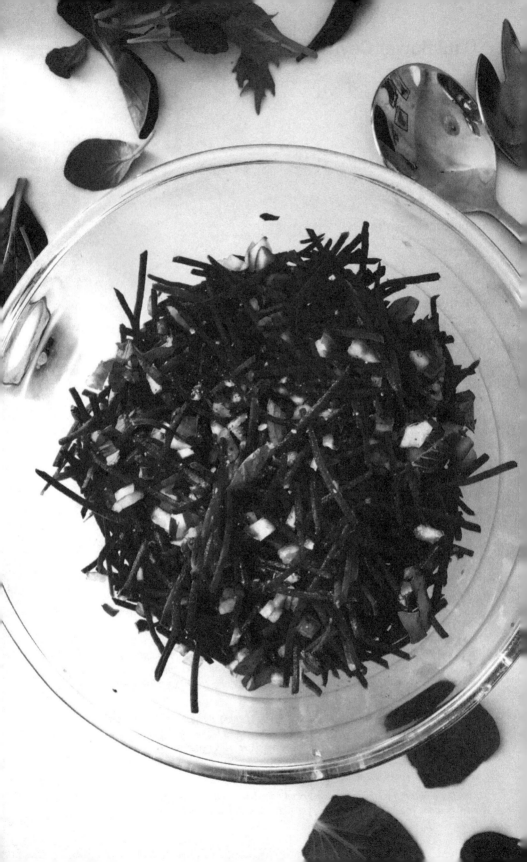

Beet Salad

Ingredients:

3 medium beets, shredded (approx. 6-7 cups)

1 large red onion, finely chopped

Green onion, chopped

½ cup balsamic vinegar

4 tsp Dijon mustard

½ tsp black pepper

Optional Additions from our Taste Testers:

Salt to taste

Grate in a carrot and/or apple for sweetness

Method:

1. Combine ingredients in a bowl and enjoy!

By Sarah Lutz

From a very young age I was constantly dealing with inflammation in various part of my body. In my teenage years I started fighting chronic fatigue, depression and the list goes on. When the summer of 2011 approached, I was diagnosed with multiple sclerosis. My symptoms continued to increase along with my need for prescription pharmaceuticals. I started to adjust my life to accommodate chronic disease. In 2014 I learned about a WFPB lifestyle and started to completely change my mindset. I quickly lost weight, got off all pharmaceutical drugs, but my pain was still holding on.

In 2018, I stumbled across Dr Goldner's work, and my life totally spiraled. In spiraled, I mean in a PHENOMENAL WAY! Participating in Dr. G's 6-Week Rapid Recovery Group was one of the BEST things I've ever done for myself. After 6 weeks, I continued the protocol on my own and within 2-3 months my pain was completely gone!

Nourishing your body with the correct foods, exercise, self-love, and mindset will 100% change your life! Kick your negativity to the curb and take care of yourself!

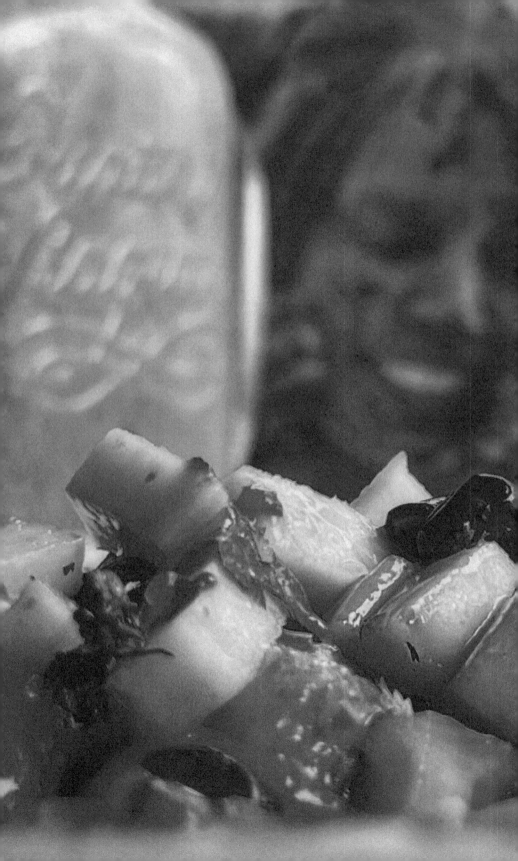

Kohlrabi Salad

Ingredients:

1 kohlrabi, in pieces

1 mango, in cubes

½ cup of fresh pineapple, diced

½ cup of pomegranate seeds

A dash of oil-free, sugar-free chili sauce

½ cup cilantro, hand chopped fresh

Salt and pepper to taste

Method:

1. Combine ingredients in a bowl.
2. Let the flavors infuse for a while, it will taste even better.

By Mirjam Letsch | @mirjamletschphotography

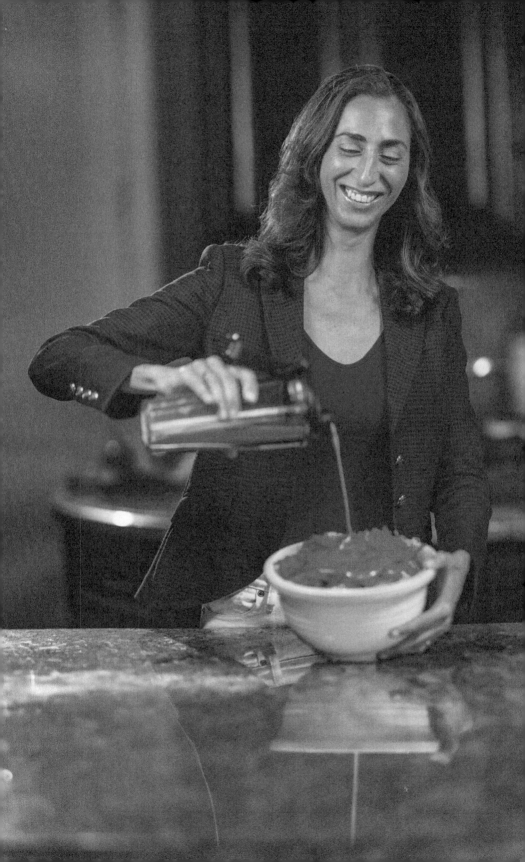

SAVORY DRESSINGS, DIPS, AND SAUCES

*I think a great sauce or dressing is
really the key to a satisfying meal.
Having the right dip, dressing or sauce
can make all of the difference!*

-Brooke Goldner, M.D.

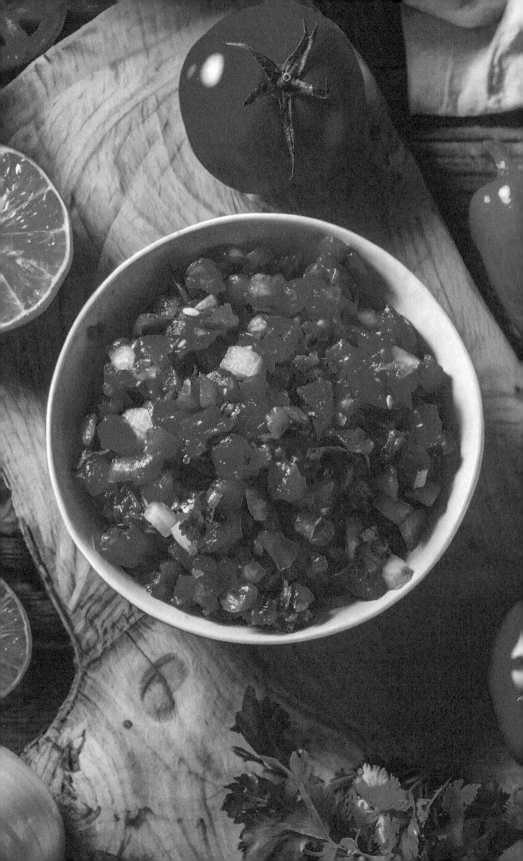

Dr. G's Pico de Gallo

Ingredients:

16 oz tomatoes, diced

1 cup diced white onion

½ cup minced fresh cilantro (about 1 bunch)

¼ cup lime juice

½ tsp salt or more to taste.

Optional:

1 jalapeño or serrano pepper, seeds removed then minced.

Instructions:

1. Add all the ingredients to a bowl and mix together. Add salt to taste.

2. Serve immediately or refrigerate to store and use the next day.

3. Use as a dressing or a dip.

By Brooke Goldner, M.D.

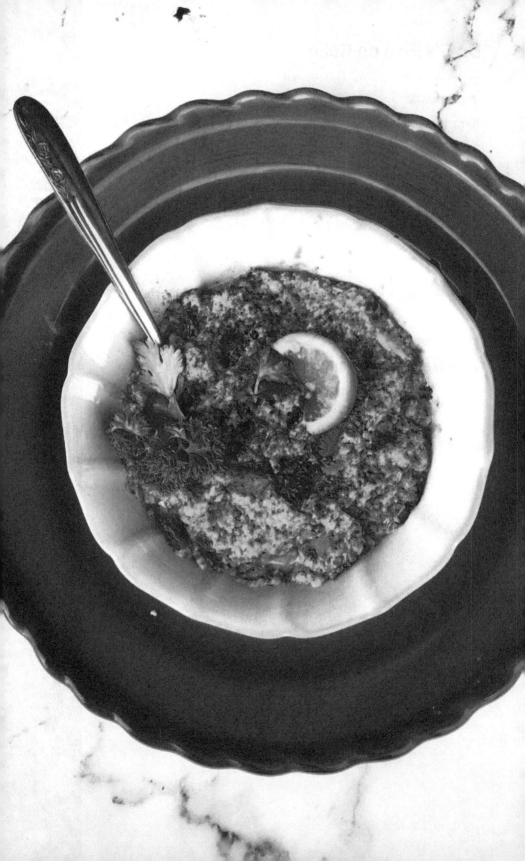

Broccomoli

Ingredients:

1-2 small avocados

1 lb fresh broccoli florets

2-4 cloves fresh garlic

¼ small red onion (or 3-4 stalks of green onion)

2 fresh squeezed limes

1 tsp ground cumin

1 TB chili powder (more to taste)

Dash of chipotle powder or cayenne to taste)

Fresh tomatoes (optional)

Cilantro (optional)

Parsley (optional)

Red bell pepper (optional)

Method:

1. Place all ingredients into a food processor and blend until you get the consistency you want for dipping. You could also blend in a high-speed blender with a little extra water to make a salad dressing.

2. Near the end of chopping (so they just get a rough chop), add your choice of the optional ingredients if desired.

By Chris Boyle

I suffered from a rare condition called AL amyloidosis, a rare disease in which a person's antibody producing cells do not function properly and results in amyloid deposits which can cause severe damage to the body's organs. In my case, this particularly affected my heart.

I had heart failure issues, low weight, shortness of breath, and stage 2 kidney disease. I then received a heart transplant that led to the remission of the amyloidosis, but I would need a follow up stem cell transplant the following year. A year later, while trying to prepare for the stem cell transplant, I found that I was extremely sensitive to anti-rejection drugs and my kidney numbers were quickly declining. I went from stage 2 kidney disease to stage 3 and was progressing to stage 4.

In the fall of 2018, I started the 6-Week Rapid Recovery Group. Within just two weeks, I went from borderline stage 4 kidney disease back to stage 3 and then back to stage 2! Since then, I have continued hyper-nourishing and describe myself as being in great health. I very much resonated with finding self care time every day and enjoy time next to my garden every morning.

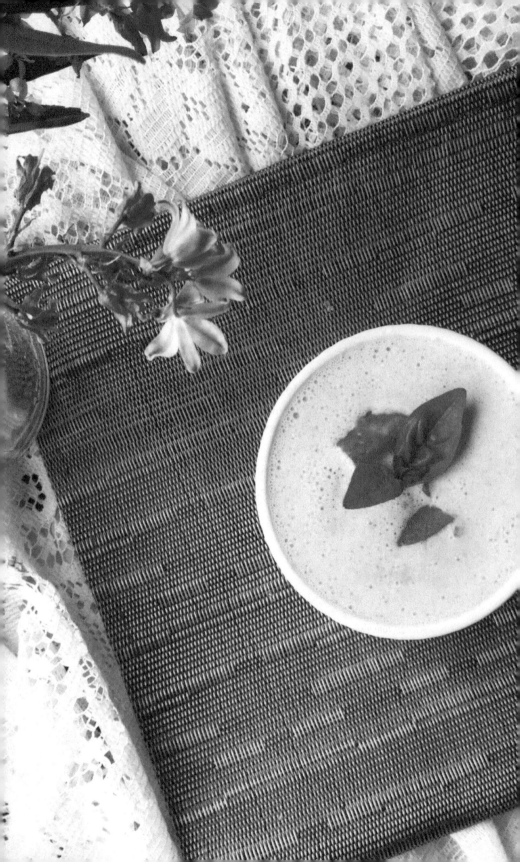

Dr. G's Citrus Salad Dressing

Ingredients:

2 TB apple cider vinegar

¼ cup water

1 tsp Braggs Liquid Aminos or salt

⅔ cup pineapple

⅔ cup mango

4 basil leaves

Method:

1. Place all ingredients in a high-speed blender in the order listed.

2. Blend until smooth.

By Brooke Goldner, M.D.

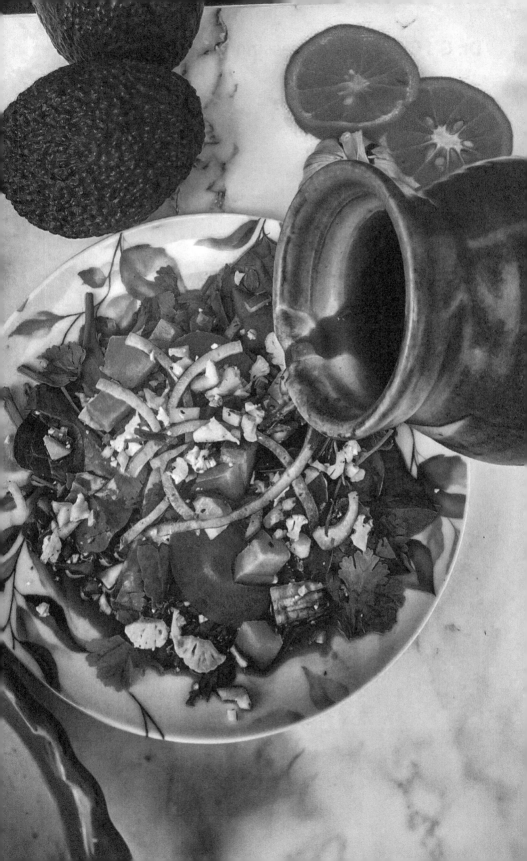

Dr. G's Garlic Ginger Dressing

Ingredients:

¼ cup Braggs Liquid Aminos

¼ cup sugar free rice vinegar

¼ cup water

¼ tsp minced fresh garlic

¼ tsp minced fresh ginger

Method:

1. Place all ingredients in a high-speed blender in the order listed.
2. Blend until smooth.

By Brooke Goldner, M.D.

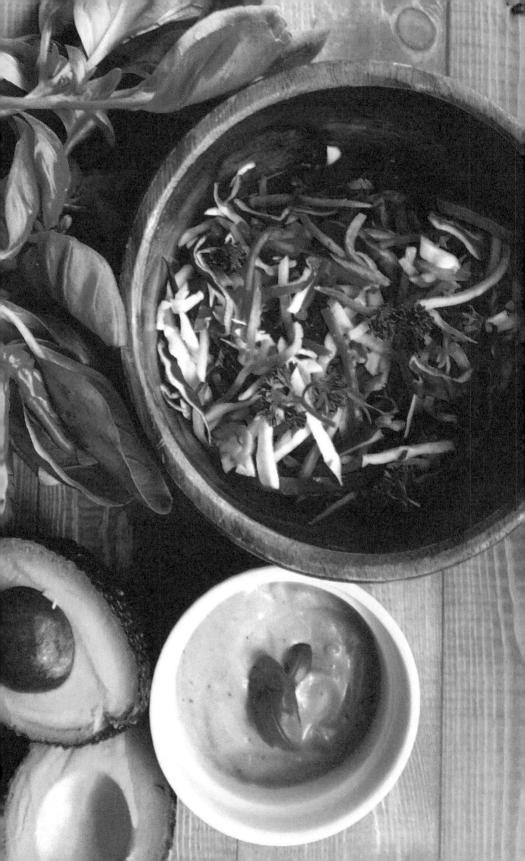

Dr. G's Tangy Avocado Dressing

Ingredients:

1 avocado

½ cup water

3 TB white vinegar

1 cup cilantro

Juice of 2 limes

Salt and pepper to taste

Method:

1. Place all ingredients in a high-speed blender

2. Blend until smooth.

By Brooke Goldner, M.D.

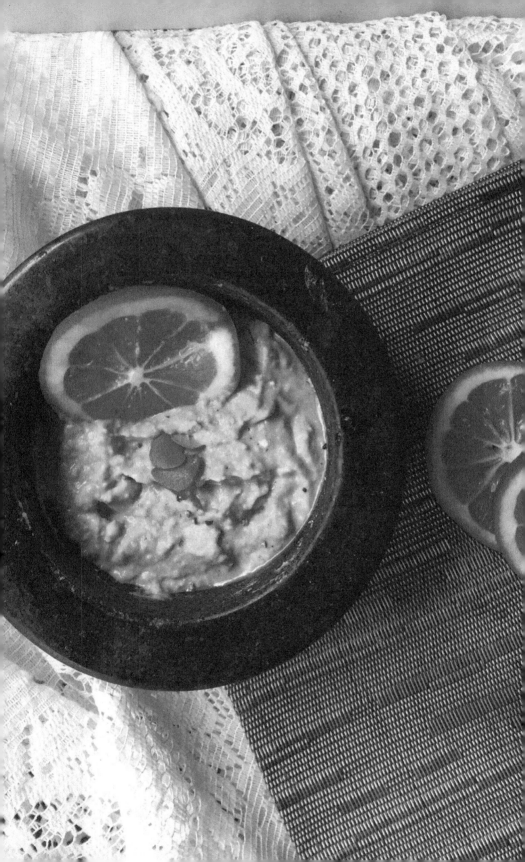

Dr. G's Simple Avocado Dressing

Ingredients:

1 avocado

½ cup water or unsweetened almond milk – more if thinner consistency desired

1 TB lemon juice

1 clove garlic

Salt and pepper to taste

Method:

1. Place all ingredients in a high-speed blender in the order listed.
2. Blend until smooth.

By Brooke Goldner, M.D.

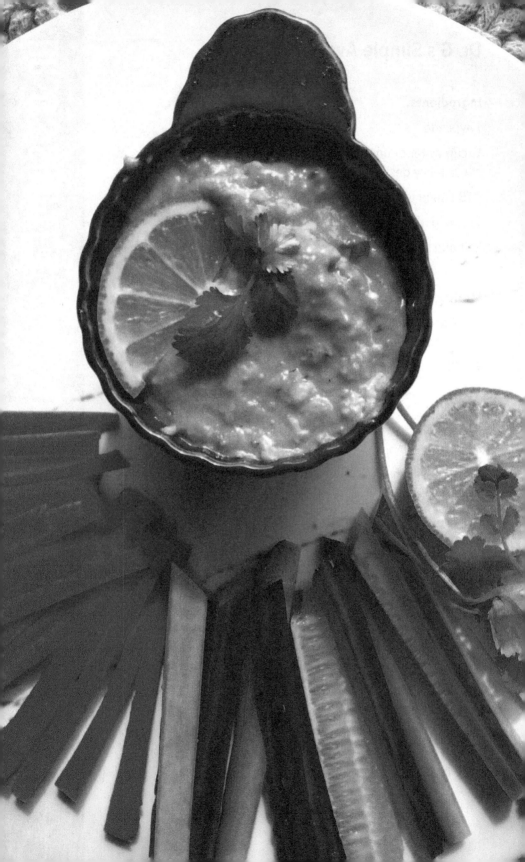

Creamy Omega-3 Veggie Dipper

Ingredients:

4 TB flax oil

1 avocado

1 lemon, juiced

1 bunch of cilantro

Salt to taste

Method:

1. Place all ingredients in a high-speed blender in the order listed.

2. Blend until smooth.

By Hilda Moleski

I struggled with deep fatigue and being overweight. I lost 13 pounds during the 6-Week Rapid Recovery Group and felt remarkably energetic by the end of the six weeks!

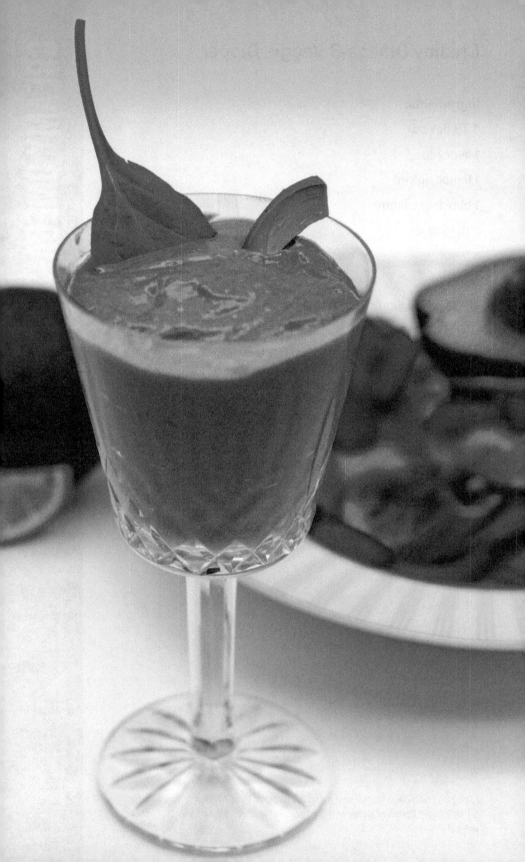

Dr. G's Avocado Caesar Salad Dressing

Kids love it!

Ingredients:

1 large avocado

3 TB lemon juice,

3 TB Braggs Liquid Aminos

2 TB Dijon mustard

3 cloves garlic

⅓ cup fortified nutritional yeast

Filtered water (about 1 ½ cups)

Method:

1. Start with about a cup of water and blend in Vitamix blender with all of the other ingredients. Slowly add water until desired consistency is reached.

2. Use what you want and store leftovers in the refrigerator. You'll need to add more water the next day as it thickens overnight.

By Brooke Goldner, M.D.

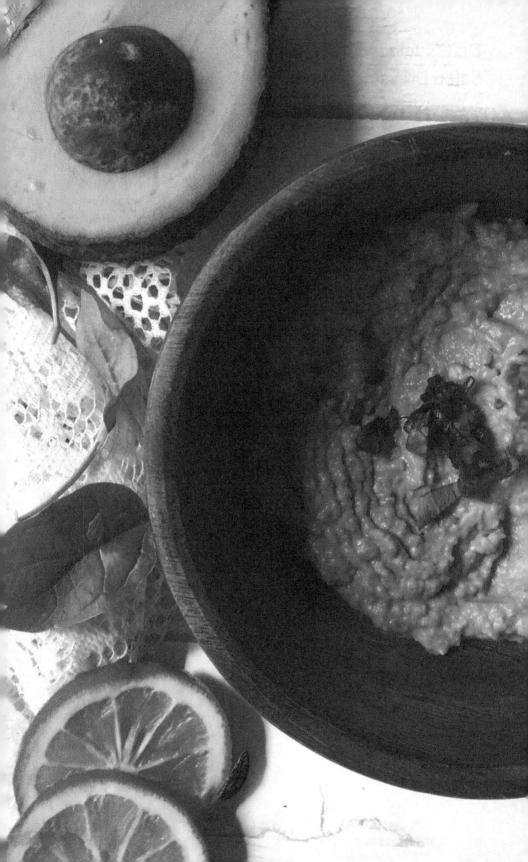

Simple Guacamole

Ingredients:

4 avocados

1 ½ limes, juiced

2 tsp onion powder

Ground black pepper to taste (optional)

Method:

1. Combine all ingredients in a bowl.

2. Mash and serve.

By Laura Rivero

I remember when I heard about Dr. Goldner through another website. I read/heard her story and started looking for more information. I finally contacted her. We scheduled a consultation phone call where I explained to her what I was going through. At the time, I had been struggling with a lot of pain. I had been diagnosed with RA, Lyme, anemia and my inflammation markers were off the charts high! Her enthusiasm is so real and nurturing that I decided to do her 6-Week Rapid Recovery Program.

The program was very eye opening. It helped me realize how and why I got to where I was. I had been neglecting myself for years! I love my family, but it's so true that to take care of others, you need to care for yourself first. The program was what I needed to get a boost into my recovery. I felt better, lost weight, which is an awesome side effect! After her program, I continued eating a plant-based diet. I am now living pain free. I want to thank you Dr. G for everything you did for me and for everything you continue to do. God bless you.

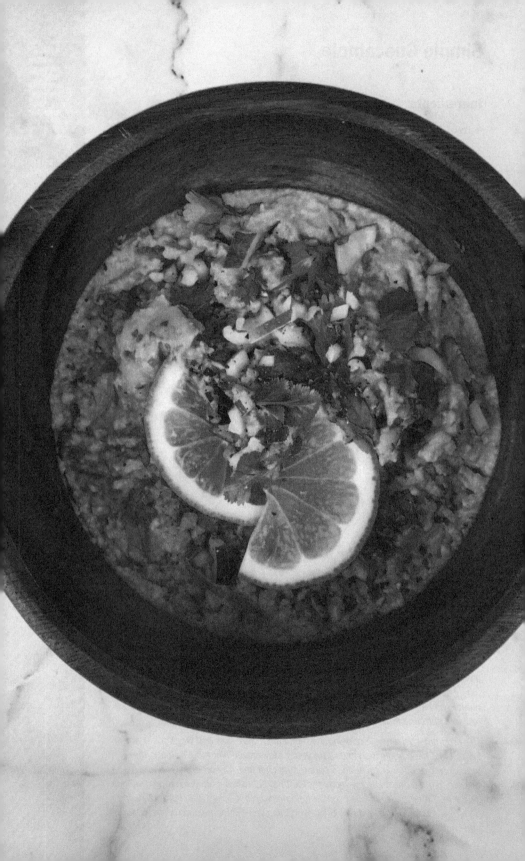

Gourmet Guacamole

Ingredients:

4 avocados

1 large lemon, juiced

½ cup red onion

¼ cup cilantro

1 large tomato, chopped

½ jalapeno, seeded and chopped (optional)

Salt to taste

Method:

1. Combine all ingredients in a bowl.
2. Mash and serve.

By Laura Rivero

I remember when I heard about Dr. Goldner through another website. I read/heard her story and started looking for more information. I finally contacted her. We scheduled a consultation phone call where I explained to her what I was going through. At the time, I had been struggling with a lot of pain. I had been diagnosed with RA, Lyme, anemia and my inflammation markers were off the charts high! Her enthusiasm is so real and nurturing that I decided to do her 6-Week Rapid Recovery Program.

The program was very eye opening. It helped me realize how and why I got to where I was. I had been neglecting myself for years! I love my family, but it's so true that to take care of others, you need to care for yourself first. The program was what I needed to get a boost into my recovery. I felt better, lost weight, which is an awesome side effect! After her program, I continued eating a plant-based diet. I am now living pain free. I want to thank you Dr. G for everything you did for me and for everything you continue to do. God bless you.

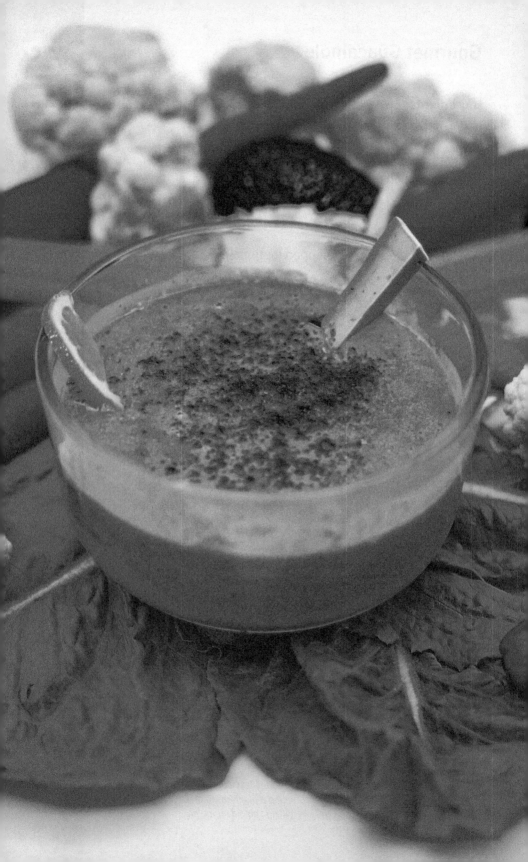

Smoky Dip

Ingredients:

½ cup water

½ cup unsweetened almond milk

2 avocados

½ cup lemon juice, fresh

1 TB nutritional yeast

1 TB minced garlic (3 cloves)

2 tsp Braggs Liquid Aminos

1 tsp salt

1 tsp chili powder

½ tsp coriander

½ tsp paprika

Method:

1. Place all ingredients in a high speed blender in the order listed.
2. Blend until smooth.

By Laurie Lynn Martin

When I first watched Dr. Goldner's free classes, I was obese, I didn't feel good physically, and I had a recent mastectomy to remove breast cancer.

I began to follow the Dr. Goldner's protocol and eventually signed up for the 6-Week Rapid Recovery Program. It really helped me see how to put all the pieces together and make even more progress.

Since then, I have lost 76 lbs, I have more energy, and I feel better physically than I ever thought possible. Thank you Dr. G!

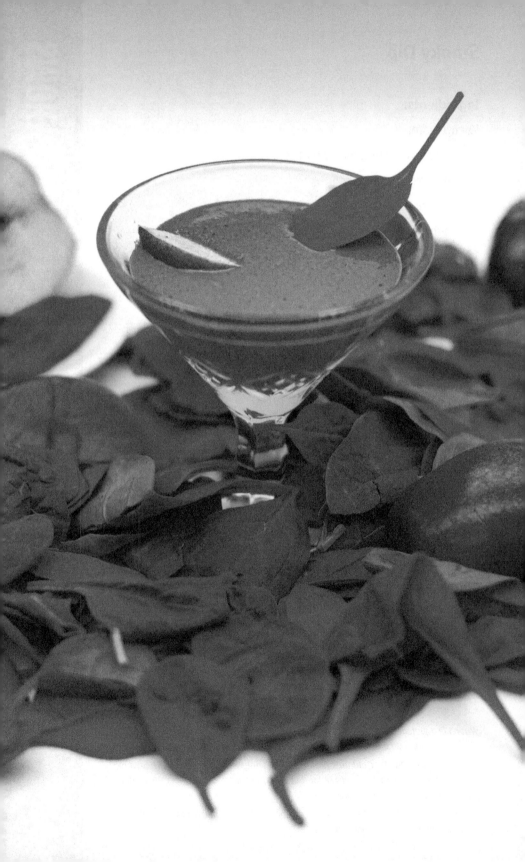

Dr. G's Cheesy Nooch Dressing

Ingredients:

1 cup nutritional yeast

½ cup Braggs Liquid Aminos

½ cup of apple cider vinegar

½ cup cold-pressed flaxseed oil or chia oil

1 clove garlic

Method:

1. Add all ingredients to your blender and blend. You can add water if you want to make it a thinner consistency.

By Brooke Goldner, M.D.

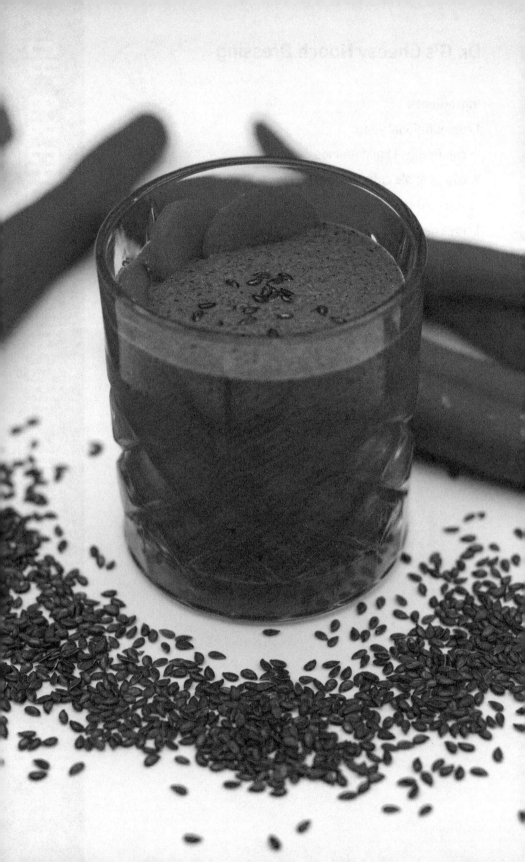

Caesar Dressing

Ingredients:

1 ½ cup water

1 ½ cup balsamic vinegar

1 cup fresh pressed carrot juice

¼ cup lemon juice

1 TB Braggs Liquid Aminos

2 TB Dijon mustard

3 cloves garlic

⅓ cup nutritional yeast

6 TB Flax

1 TB Mrs. Dash

½ TB onion powder

½ TB garlic powder

2 tsp Benson's Table Tasty

¼ tsp cayenne

Method:

1. Combine all ingredients in a blender and blend until smooth and creamy.

By Sarah Lutz

From a very young age I was constantly dealing with inflammation in various part of my body. In my teenage years I started fighting chronic fatigue, depression and the list goes on. When the summer of 2011 approached, I was diagnosed with multiple sclerosis. My symptoms continued to increase along with my need for prescription pharmaceuticals. I started to adjust my life to accommodate chronic disease. In 2014 I learned about a WFPB lifestyle and started to completely change my mindset. I quickly lost weight, got off all pharmaceutical drugs, but my pain was still holding on.

In 2018, I stumbled across Dr Goldner's work, and my life totally spiraled. In spiraled, I mean in a PHENOMENAL WAY! Participating in Dr. G's 6-Week Rapid Recovery Group was one of the BEST things I've ever done for myself. After 6 weeks, I continued the protocol on my own and within 2-3 months my pain was completely gone!

Nourishing your body with the correct foods, exercise, self-love, and mindset will 100% change your life! Kick your negativity to the curb and take care of yourself!

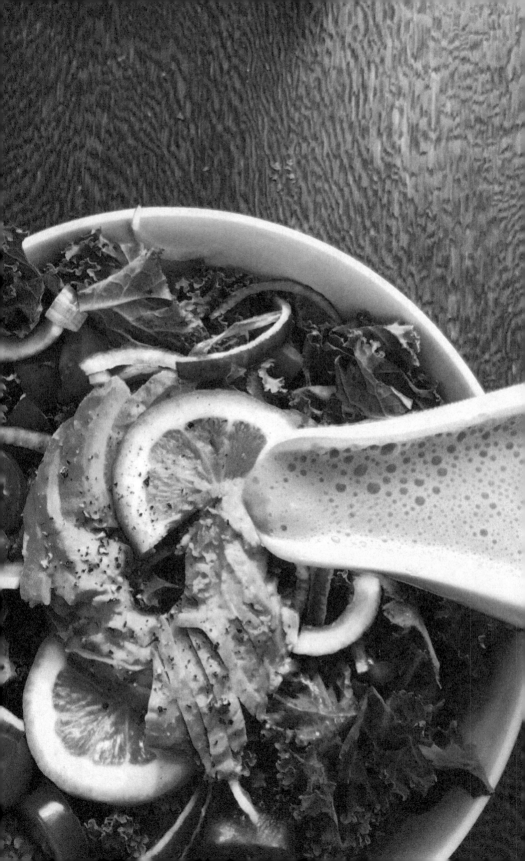

Carrot Ginger Dressing

Ingredients:

1 ¼ cup fresh pressed carrot juice

¼ cup white balsamic vinegar

1 clove garlic

½ TB garlic powder

½ inch fresh ginger

4 ½ TB flax seed

½ TB crushed red pepper

Method:

1. Place carrot juice, white balsamic vinegar, and flax seed into high powered blender. Blend until flax seeds are almost fully blended.

2. Add remaining ingredients and blend until smooth and creamy.

By Sarah Lutz

From a very young age I was constantly dealing with inflammation in various part of my body. In my teenage years I started fighting chronic fatigue, depression and the list goes on. When the summer of 2011 approached, I was diagnosed with multiple sclerosis. My symptoms continued to increase along with my need for prescription pharmaceuticals. I started to adjust my life to accommodate chronic disease. In 2014 I learned about a WFPB lifestyle and started to completely change my mindset. I quickly lost weight, got off all pharmaceutical drugs, but my pain was still holding on.

In 2018, I stumbled across Dr Goldner's work, and my life totally spiraled. In spiraled, I mean in a PHENOMENAL WAY! Participating in Dr. G's 6-Week Rapid Recovery Group was one of the BEST things I've ever done for myself. After 6 weeks, I continued the protocol on my own and within 2-3 months my pain was completely gone!

Nourishing your body with the correct foods, exercise, self-love, and mindset will 100% change your life! Kick your negativity to the curb and take care of yourself!

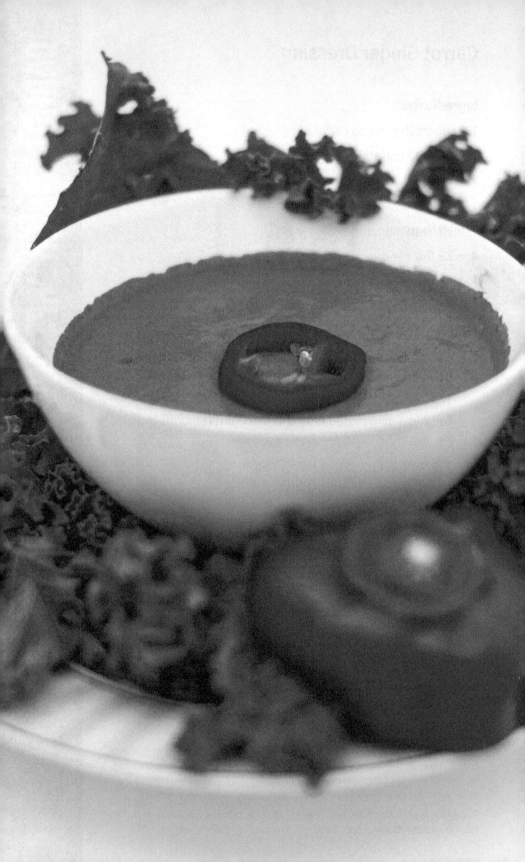

Holly's Spicy Pepper Dressing

Ingredients:

1 bell pepper, cut into large pieces

6 TB flaxseed oil

3 TB vinegar (red wine or apple cider)

1 TB Dijon mustard

2 tsp onion powder

1-2 tsp chia seeds

1 tsp mushroom umami seasoning (optional)

Cayenne pepper and black pepper to taste (optional)

Method:

1. Put all ingredients into a blender and serve over a giant salad!

By Holly Herzog, MS, RD, LDN

I have been living with a Crohn's Disease diagnosis for 16 years now and have never felt more confident in how to treat it. As a dietitian, I know that "food heals" and I have been able to experience that in full force in the 6-Week Rapid Recovery Group program. On top of the foods, I also have learned the importance of self-care, self-talk, forgiveness, meditation, and sleep. I am doing so much better now. Sometimes I slip and fall, but I know what to do now when I get back up. I have gained a wealth of knowledge through the 6-Week Rapid Recovery Program and will be forever grateful.

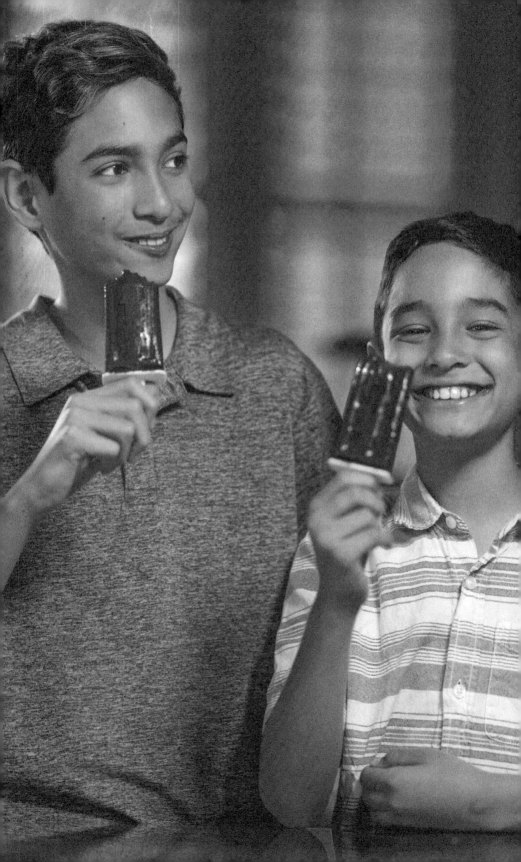

HEALTHY
DESSERTS

You can totally satisfy your craving for something sweet without sabotaging your health. I included some of my favorite sweet treats, and my Rapid Recovery graduates added some drool-worthy recipes that will keep you coming back for more!

– Brooke Goldner, M.D.

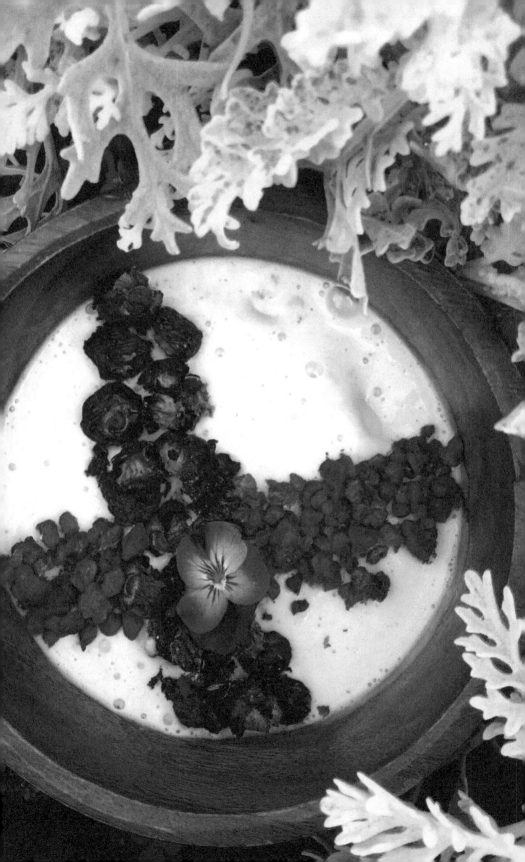

Dr. G's Dreamy Banana Guilt-Free Ice Cream

Ingredients:

4 frozen Bananas (frozen at least 48 hours so they are fully solid)

1 splash unsweetened almond milk

Requires a high powered blender.

Method:

1. Break up the bananas into quarters and put into your Vitamix blender. Add the unsweetened almond milk and cover.

2. Blend on high using the tamper to mash the bananas down towards to blade. Blend until smooth, about 30 seconds. Serve and eat immediately – melts fast!

3. You can add cacao powder, or other fruits like strawberries or blueberries to make different flavors.

By Brooke Goldner, M.D.

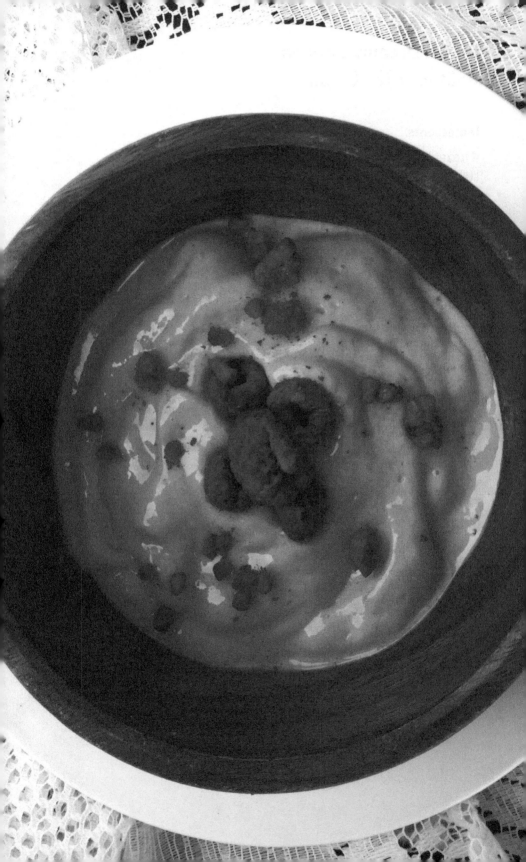

Cauliflower Carrot Banana Ice Cream

Ingredients:

½ cup unsweetened vanilla almond milk

2 cup fresh cauliflower

¾ cup frozen carrot

2 small-medium frozen banana

1 tsp pumpkin pie spice

½ tsp Ceylon cinnamon

Method:

1. Place all ingredients in a high powered blender and process until thick and smooth.

2. Scoop into bowls and serve with a sprinkle of cinnamon and extra fruit.

By Sarah Lutz

From a very young age I was constantly dealing with inflammation in various part of my body. In my teenage years I started fighting chronic fatigue, depression and the list goes on. When the summer of 2011 approached, I was diagnosed with multiple sclerosis. My symptoms continued to increase along with my need for prescription pharmaceuticals. I started to adjust my life to accommodate chronic disease. In 2014 I learned about a WFPB lifestyle and started to completely change my mindset. I quickly lost weight, got off all pharmaceutical drugs, but my pain was still holding on.

In 2018, I stumbled across Dr Goldner's work, and my life totally spiraled. In spiraled, I mean in a PHENOMENAL WAY! Participating in Dr. G's 6-Week Rapid Recovery Group was one of the BEST things I've ever done for myself. After 6 weeks, I continued the protocol on my own and within 2-3 months my pain was completely gone!

Nourishing your body with the correct foods, exercise, self-love, and mindset will 100% change your life! Kick your negativity to the curb and take care of yourself!

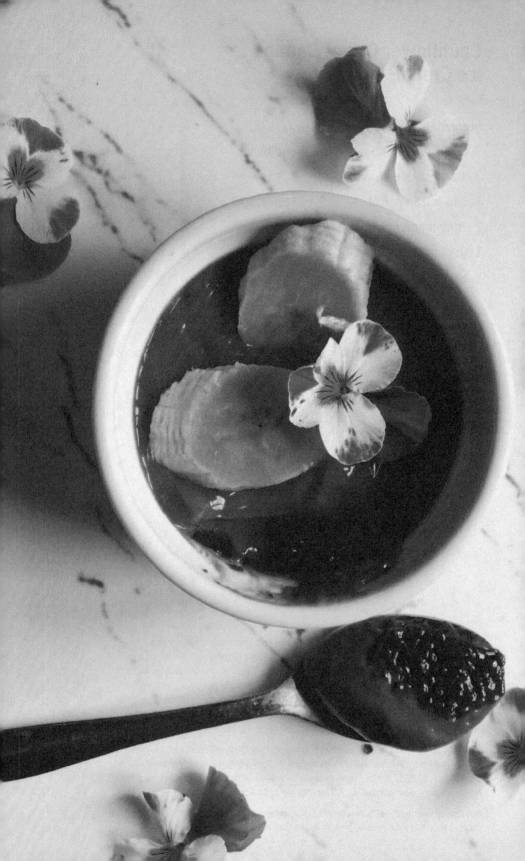

Chocolate Frosted Raspberry Dessert

Ingredients:

¼ cup frozen raspberries   1 TB cacao

2 TB flaxseeds   2-3 TB water

½ banana

Method:

1. Thaw and mash the frozen raspberries.

2. Grind the flaxseeds in a small coffee grinder and add to the raspberries with 2 - 3 tablespoons of water.

3. Stir and put in the fridge to set up. I like it thicker than pudding so it's nice and sturdy to hold the "frosting."

4. In a separate bowl, mash the banana and mix it with the cacao.

5. Put the banana mixture in the fridge until ready to eat, and then spread the banana mix on top of the raspberry and flax mixture.

By Janice Dickson

In the 6-Week Rapid Recovery Group, I learned how to incorporate all parts of the protocol...food, sleep, water, exercise, self care, joy, and problem solving. I began the group with stiff, painful shoulders and elbows and very limited range of motion. I could not reach over my head or behind my back. I experienced pain and burning when my hands and fingers were exposed to cold or frozen things. My myasthenia symptoms were droopy eyelids, double vision, and muscle weakness. My gait was unsteady and staggering. I also experienced severe pain in my upper back and diaphragm after prolonged standing.

At the end of the six weeks, my hands were no longer sensitive to cold. I could put my hands behind my back at waist level, touch the back of my neck and raise my arms with much less pain. My eyelids no longer drooped and I was walking like a normal person. I could stand without needing to take a break to lay down to relieve the pain.

Today I still continues smoothies and plant based eating, and I have maintained my results. I now have no shoulder/elbow pain and I have a very good range of motion as long as I don't stray into vegan junk food or oils.

I am forever grateful to Brooke and Thomas for the care and teaching I received in the group. It was a wonderful experience.

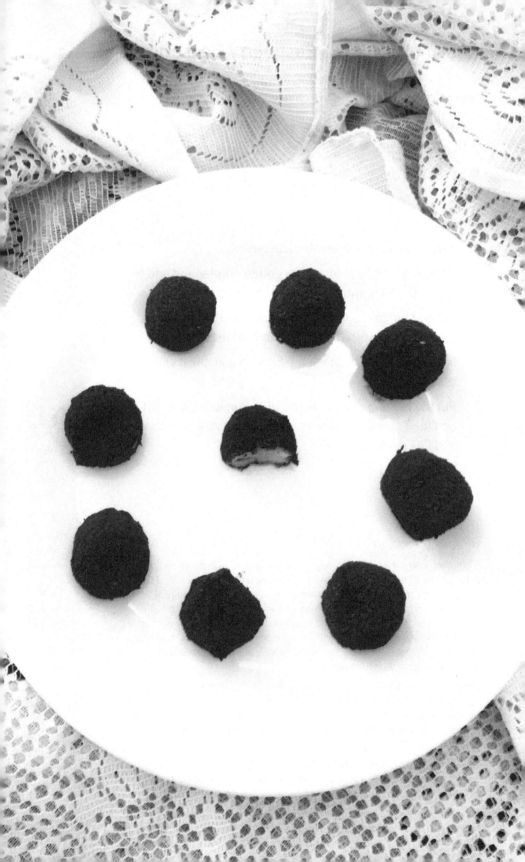

Dr. G's Easy Raw Macaroons

Makes 4-5 balls

Ingredients:

1 banana

¼ cup cacao

Method:

1. Mash a banana with a fork and roll into 1" balls

2. Roll each banana ball in cacao powder.

3. Refrigerate for at least 2 hours or overnight to firm up.

Recipe note: If you have a dehydrator you can dehydrate for an hour to make outside crispy before refrigerating.

By Brooke Goldner, M.D.

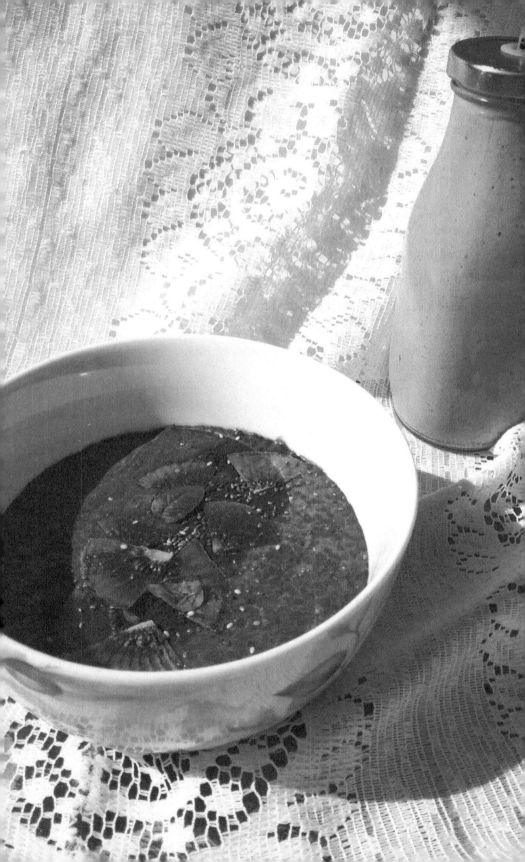

Dr. G's Chocolate Chia Seed Pudding

Ingredients:

2 TB chia seeds

½ cup unsweetened almond milk

1 TB cacao powder

½ tsp vanilla extract

1 ripe banana (with brown spots on the skin)

Method:

1. Stir or whisk all the ingredients together and leave on countertop for 20 minutes. (To optimize omega-3 absorption, blend the mixture to break up the seeds).

2. Stir again after 20 minutes so cacao dissolves.

3. Refrigerate 4-6 hours or overnight to thicken.

4. When ready to serve, slice up banana and mix into pudding.

By Brooke Goldner, M.D.

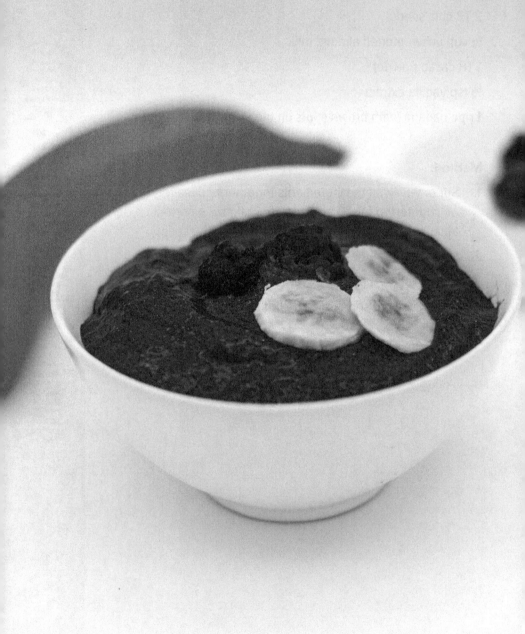

Cacao Berry Chia Pudding

Ingredients:

¼ cup chia seeds

1 very ripe medium size banana

1 TB cacao

1 cup unsweetened almond milk

½ cup Blueberries and/or raspberries

Method:

1. In a high powered blender, blend chia seeds, banana, unsweetened almond milk, and cacao powder.

2. Refrigerate mixture for at least one hour.

3. Add your favorite berries right before serving and enjoy!

Recipe note: *If you don't have a high powered blender, pulse the chia seeds in a coffee grinder first, then add to the blender with the banana and almond milk mixture.*

By Anonymous

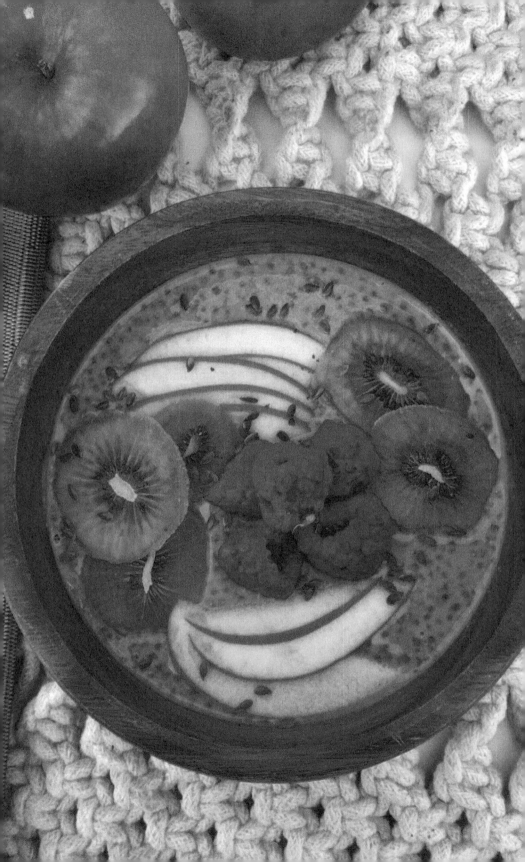

Chia Pudding

Ingredients:

1 cup unsweetened almond milk

⅛ cup chia seeds

1 ¼ TB cacao powder

½ tsp vanilla extract

½ cup mixed berries of your choice

Dash of cinnamon to taste

Method:

1. Add unsweetened almond milk, chia seeds, cacao, cinnamon and vanilla extract, to your blender and blend it until smooth.

2. Top it with some sweet berries or other fruit to serve.

By Marte Hove

I had lupus nephritis stage 4 before starting the 6-Week Rapid Recovery Program. Fatigue was my big problem and concern, not being able to do the normal things but having to be selective in my activities was hard and frustrating.

After I did the 6-Week Rapid Recovery Program back in 2018, I become free from fatigue, that was a big relief and my kidneys improved dramatically. It's now been 5 years since I participated in the group, with no flare ups and my rheumatologist classifies my lupus as in remission.

Today I still do my 64oz daily smoothie and am eating a whole food plant-based diet.

Thanks to Dr. Goldner I no longer have concerns about flare-ups and fatigue.

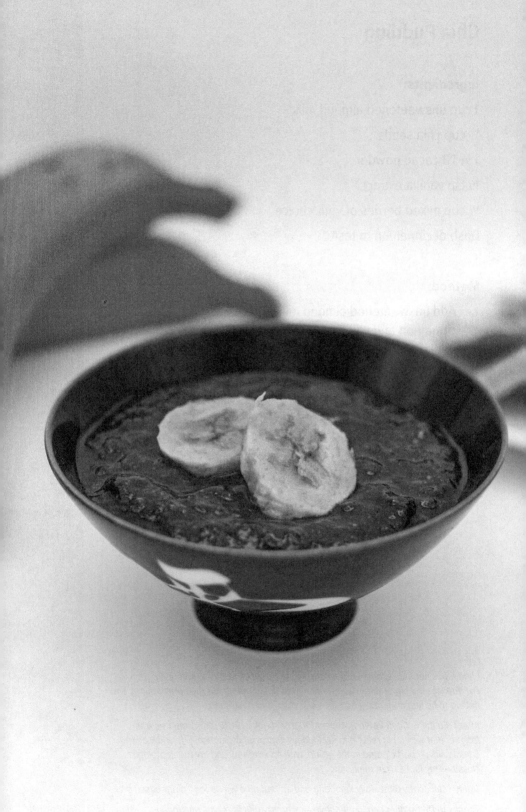

Alex's Chocolate Pudding

Ingredients:

1 large banana

1 TB cacao powder

Sprinkle of salt (optional)

Method:

1. Mash the banana with a fork (or blend it) and mix in the cacao powder. Add salt if desired.

2. Eat right away or refrigerate to eat later.

By Alex Tadlock

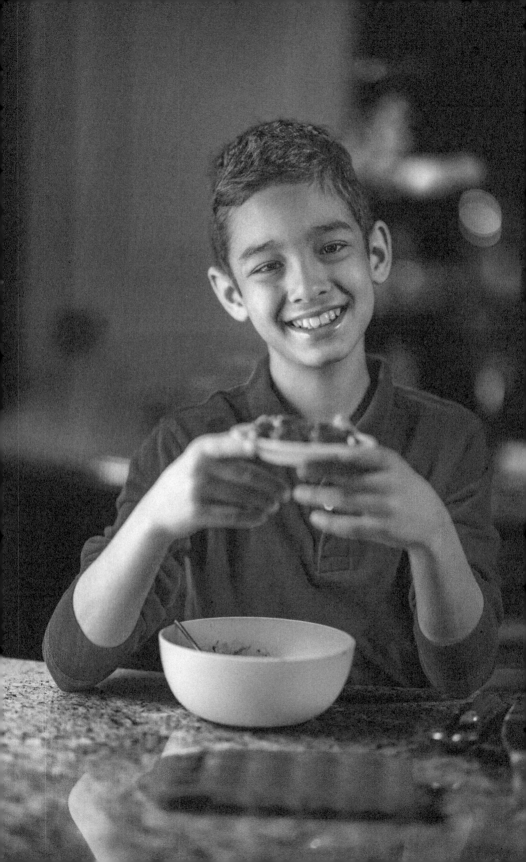

Alex's Famous Chocolate Candy Bites

Ingredients:

1 large banana

1 TB cacao powder

Sprinkle of salt (optional)

Method:

1. Mash or blend the banana with the cacao powder. Add salt if desired.

2. Pour the mixture into ice cube tray or silicone candy molds. Freeze until solid. Enjoy guilt free candy!

By Alex Tadlock

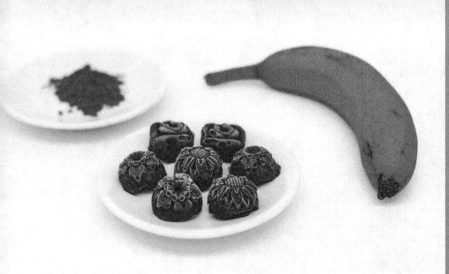

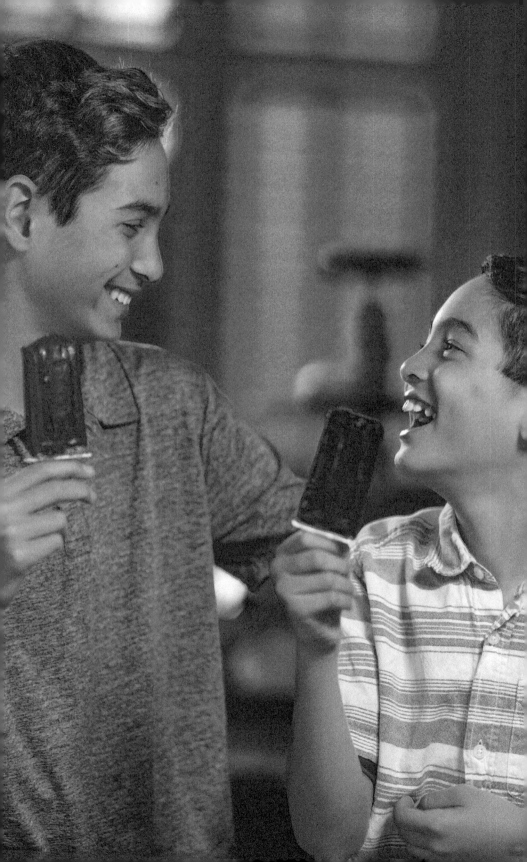

Elizabeth & Emilie's Fudge Pops

Ingredients:

3 ripe bananas

2 TB cacao powder

1 tsp vanilla extract

½ cup unsweetened almond milk

Method:

1. Blend all ingredients together well

2. Pour into popsicle molds and freeze.

By Elizabeth Enright

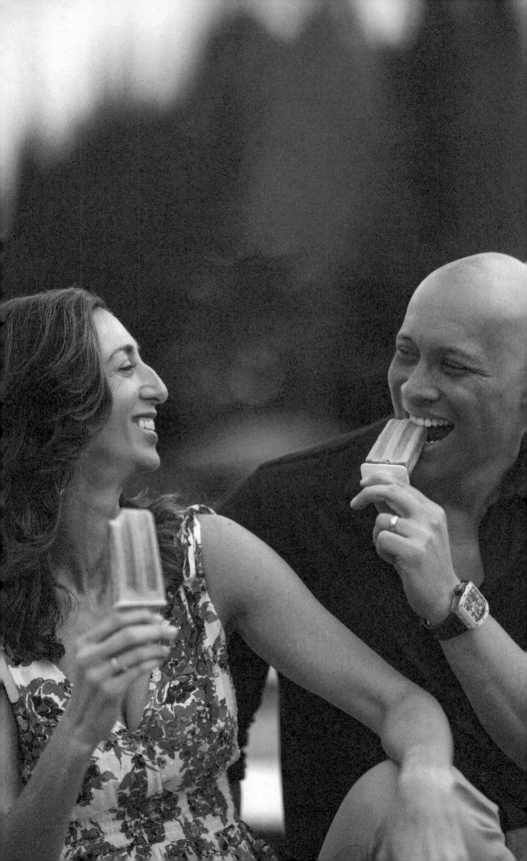

Dr. G's Mango Creamsicle Pop

Ingredients:

5 oz frozen mango

1 ½ cups unsweetened almond milk

1 banana

1 tsp vanilla extract

Method:

1. Blend up the ingredients until smooth.
2. Freeze and enjoy!

By Brooke Goldner, M.D.

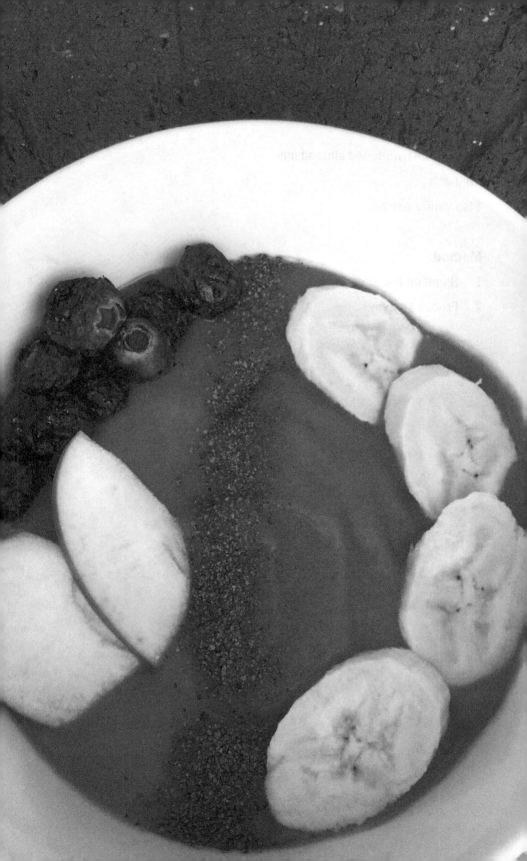

Sweet Potato Pudding

Ingredients:

16 oz raw sweet potatoes, peeled and diced, measures 3 ½ cups

1 tsp grated orange zest

1 orange, juiced (about 3 TB)

Dash of cinnamon and nutmeg to taste

2 bananas to sweeten

Dash salt (optional)

Method:

1. Place all in blender and blend, poking down or scraping blender as necessary.
2. Serve with extra banana and a sprinkling of orange zest.

Recipe note: *This recipe is like a sweet potato pudding, you can add some diced fresh pineapple into the pureed dish before serving.*

By Susan Resig

I have taught cooking for over 30 years, but struggled with autoimmune problems. I worked with Dr. Goldner in her 6-Week Rapid Recovery Group and found that the more raw my diet, the better I felt. It's been 3 years since following the 6-Week Rapid Recovery Program, and I still have more energy and radiate health at the age of 61.

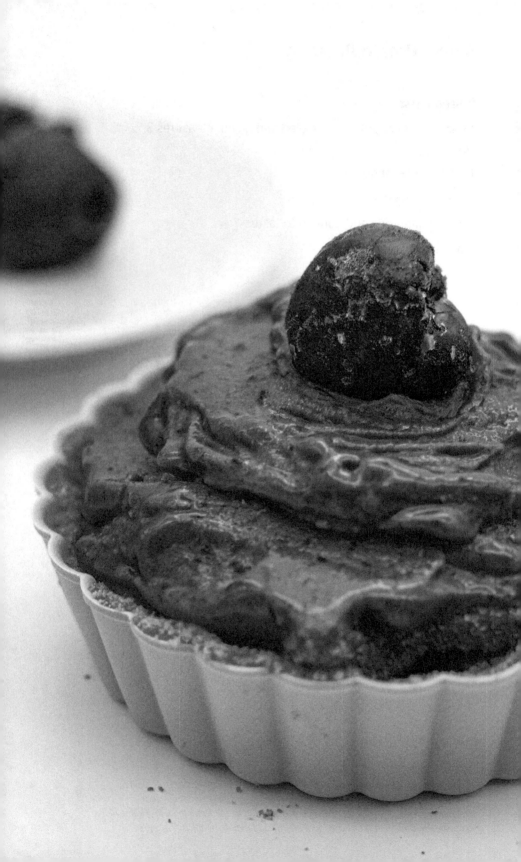

Cherry Pie

Crust Ingredients:

¼ cup flaxseeds

Pinch of salt

Dash of cinnamon

Pie Filling Ingredients:

6 oz frozen cherries and bananas

Splash unsweetened almond milk

Optional dash of vanilla extract to taste

Method:

1. Pulse flaxseeds in a coffee grinder until they are well ground. Mix in the salt and cinnamon and press into a bowl or a 4" to 6" mini-pie pan.

2. Blend the filling ingredients in a high-powered blender like a Vitamix and use the tamper to push the frozen fruit into the blade through the tamper hole in the Vitamix lid. Alternatively, you can use a frozen fruit soft serve machine.

3. Scoop the filling on to the crust and serve immediately or freeze. If you freeze it, it may need to thaw 10-15 minutes to be soft enough to eat.

Contributed By Elizabeth Wright

Original recipe by a member of our #SmoothieShred Facebook group, Leah Lapointe, who wants you to know that she was pain-free in 3 days from chronic Rheumatoid Arthritis following the Goodbye Lupus Protocol!

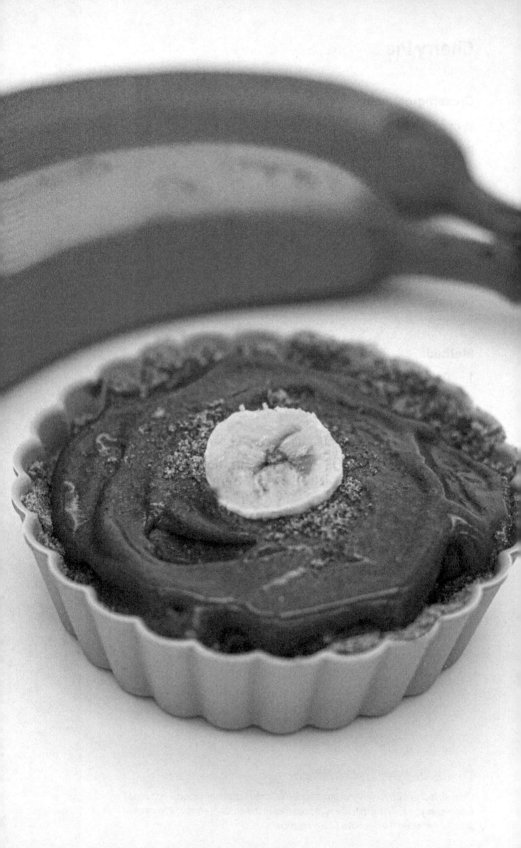

Chocolate Cream Pie

Crust Ingredients:

¼ cup flaxseeds

Pinch of salt

Dash of cinnamon

Pie Filling Ingredients:

6-8 oz frozen bananas

Splash of unsweetened almond milk

2 tsp cacao

Optional dash of vanilla extract to taste

Method:

1. Pulse flaxseeds in a coffee grinder until they are well ground. Mix in the salt and cinnamon and press into a bowl or a 4 to 6" mini-pie pan.

2. Blend the filling ingredients in a high-powered blender like a Vitamix and use the tamper to push the frozen fruit into the blade through the tamper hole in the Vitamix lid. Alternatively you can use a frozen fruit soft serve machine.

3. Scoop the filling on to the crust and serve immediately or freeze. If you freeze it, it may need to thaw 10-15 minutes to be soft enough to eat.

By Emile DeVasher

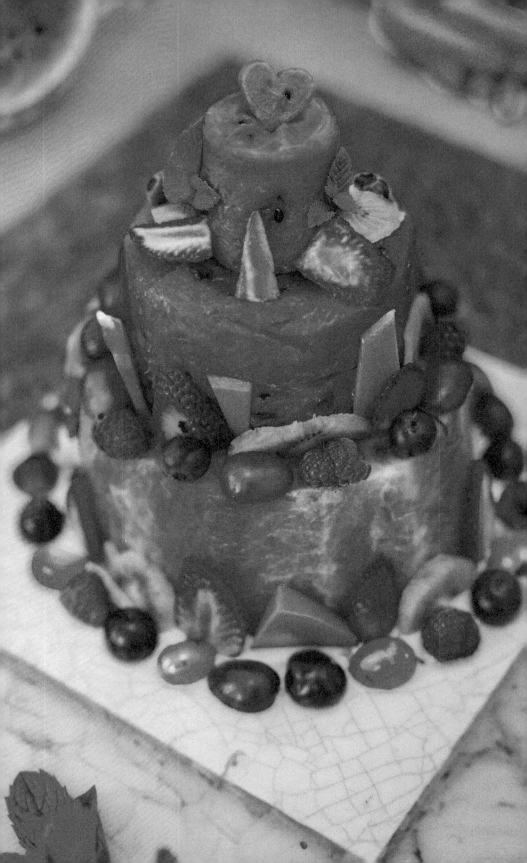

Watermelon Celebration Cake

Ingredients:

1 watermelon (or melon of your choice)

1 cup strawberries

1 cup sliced mango

1 cup grapes

Mint leaves

Optional - any fresh fruit you have!

Method:

1. Cut the watermelon ends off and then carefully remove the rind from all sides.

2. Next, cut the watermelon cylinder into 3 smaller slices (about same width - see photo).

3. Trim the sides to make round shape. You can use different sized bowls as a guide if you really want perfectly round sections.

4. Assemble the slices with largest layer on the bottom and smaller going up like a layered cake.

5. Insert toothpicks into the cake layers so that the cake stays together.

6. Time to get creative! Decorate with mint leaves and fruit listed above or any fresh fruit you like. You can use toothpicks as needed to hold pieces onto cake.

Recipe notes: For a fun option, add some pieces of Alex's Famous Chocolate Candy Bites (page 145) to add a decadent chocolate cake topper!

Another fun option: You don't need to stick with watermelon! You can make layers with honeydew melon, and cantaloupe too for a multicolored cake, or one that is made of any melon you prefer.

Note: I recommend you cut and prepare the fruit in advance and refrigerate the ingredients until it's time for cake. Then assemble it all when you are ready to serve it. If you assemble it early, it might be hard to fit into your refrigerator!

By Brooke Goldner, M.D.

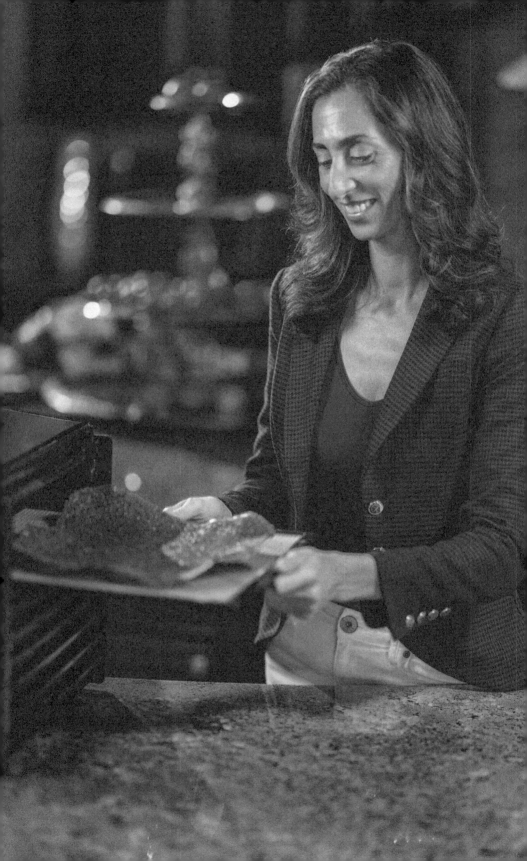

DEHYDRATED
GOODIES

You can enjoy healing on a raw vegan nutrition plan without a dehydrator, but getting one can add a lot of fun variety to your meals. Dehydrated snacks are available at stores but they often are very pricey. A dehydrator is easy to use and makes these foods readily available for a fraction of the cost.

— Brooke Goldner, M.D.

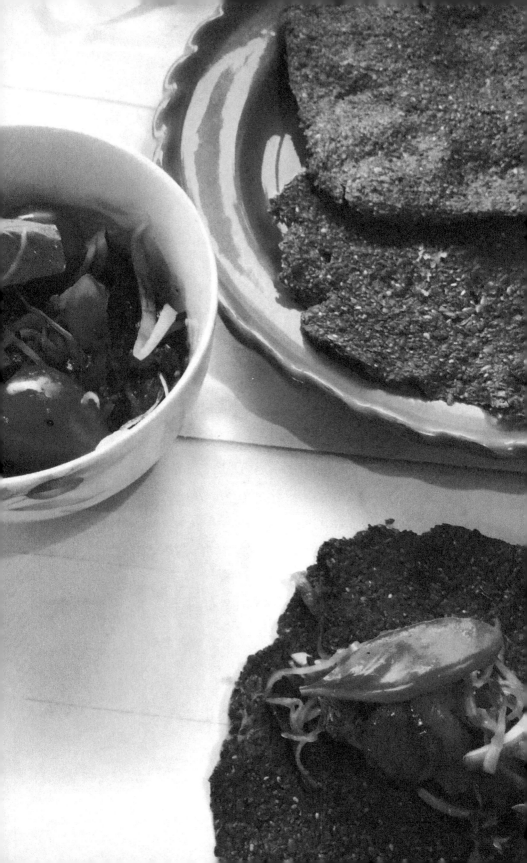

Dr. G's Tomato Flax Tortillas

Makes 8 tortillas

Ingredients:

½ cup flaxseeds

½ cup water

2 cups chopped organic tomatoes (about 2 medium tomatoes)

1 TB Braggs Liquid Aminos

Method:

1. Grind the flax seeds coarsely (I used coffee grinder)

2. Put ground seeds into your blender with 1/2 cup of water and soak for 15 minutes

3. Add the rest of the ingredients to your blender and process on high until smooth. Should be thick.

4. Pour the mixture into four (roughly) 7" circles about 1/4" thick on each Teflon sheet and dehydrate at 105F for about 1 hour, or until the top of the tortilla is dry to the touch.

5. Gently flip over each Teflon sheet and replace onto the dehydrator tray.

6. Carefully peel off the Teflon very slowly, leaving the tortillas on the dehydrator tray.

7. Put the tortillas back in the dehydrator for another 30-60 minutes, checking for the tortilla to just barely be dry to the touch, but still soft and flexible.

8. Now wrap away! Can be stored in your refrigerator. To store, lay flat between pieces of parchment paper for best results.

By Brooke Goldner, M.D.

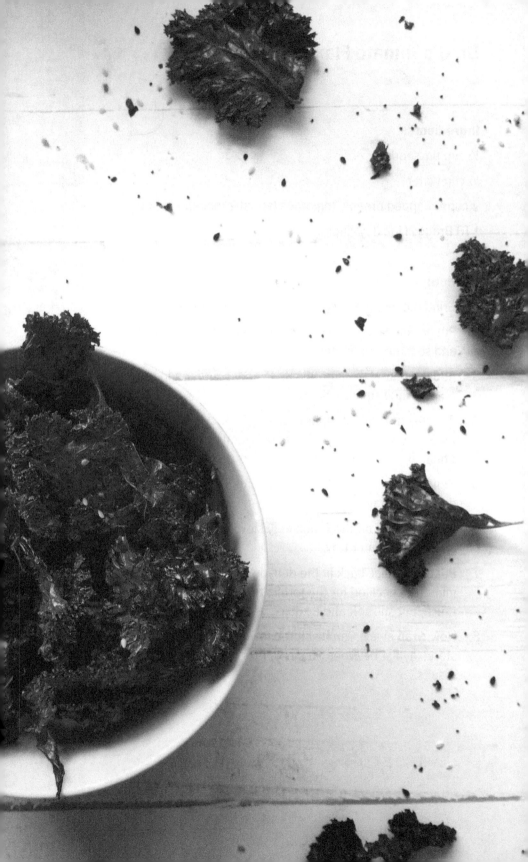

Dr. G's Crunchy Kale Chips

Ingredients:

2 bunches of kale, rinse and remove stem

1 TB apple cider vinegar

Sea salt to taste

¼ cup of nutritional yeast (more or less to taste)

Method:

1. Mix the apple cider vinegar, salt, and yeast in a large mixing bowl.

2. Tear, or roughly chop the kale leaves up into chip size pieces. Add the kale to the bowl and massage the vinegar mixture into it.

3. Spread kale out on dehydrator trays.

4. Dehydrate 5-6 hours at 115 degrees until completely dry and crunchy.

5. If you do not have a dehydrator, lay the kale out on mesh, and leave outside in a sunny location for 4-6 hours to dry.

6. Serve immediately, Store remaining kale chips in a glass jar, eat within 2 days.

By Brooke Goldner, M.D.

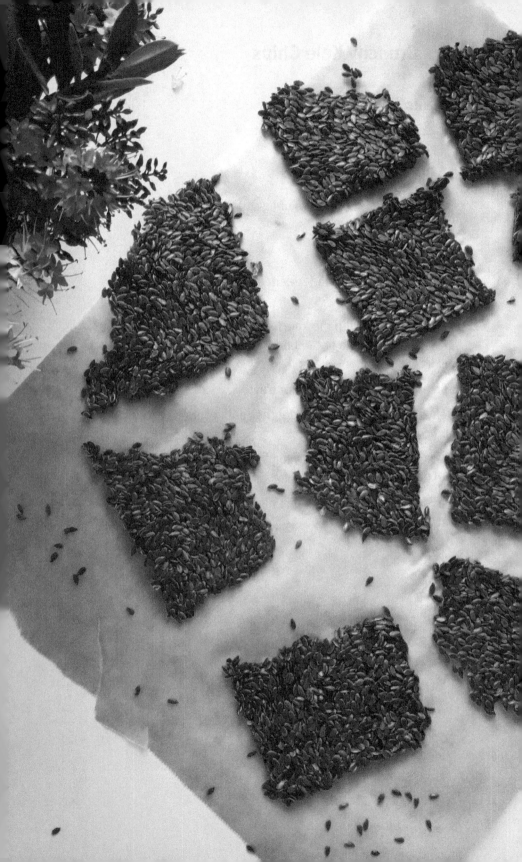

Dr. G's Super Easy Flaxseed Crackers

Ingredients:

2 cups flaxseeds

1 cup of water

½ cup Braggs Liquid Aminos (or use salt to taste)

Method:

1. Mix all ingredients in a bowl and let the bowl sit until the seeds absorb all the water and becomes a gel.

2. Line your dehydrator trays with Teflon sheets.

3. Use a spatula to spread a thin layer of flaxseed gel on each sheet, about 1-2 mm thick.

4. Place trays into the dehydrator set to 115 degrees.

5. Check every couple hours. When the top of the crackers are dry to the touch, turn them over and remove the Teflon sheet to finish drying.

6. Total drying time is usually around 12 hours, although you should check on them regularly and remove them when they easy break and are dry inside.

Recipe Tip: You can substitute chia seeds for some or all of the flaxseeds if you prefer or have an allergy to flax.

Healing Tip: These don't count towards your total omega-3 for the day, just consider them a free crunchy snack!

By Brooke Goldner, M.D.

DR. G'S SUPER EASY FLAXSEED CRACKERS

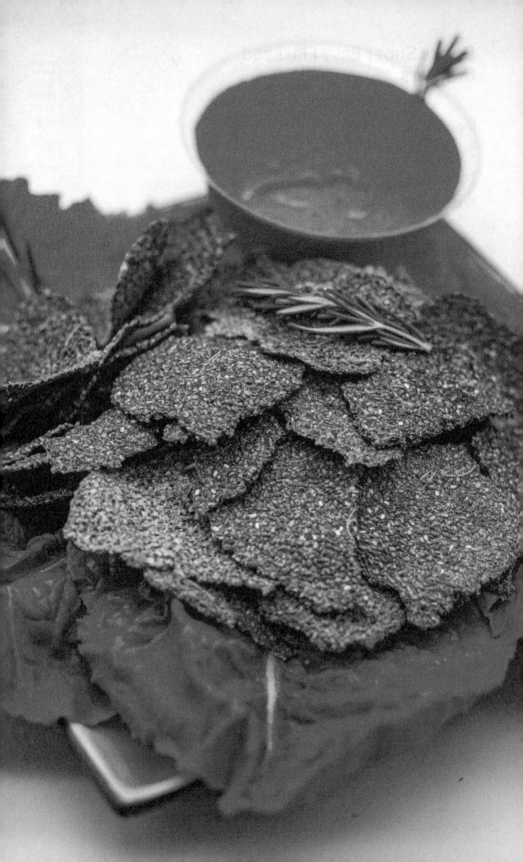

Low Histamine Chia Chips

This recipe makes about 24 chips.

Ingredients:

½ cup chia seeds

1 ½ cup water

½ tsp salt

1 tsp apple cider vinegar

1 tsp fresh rosemary

Method:

1. Put all ingredients in a bowl except the chia seeds.

2. Stir half of the chia seeds into the bowl.

3. Grind the other half of the chia seeds, add it to the bowl and stir again.

4. Stir every few minutes until it becomes a thick goo, maybe 20 minutes or more.

5. Spread mixture thinly on a Teflon dehydrator sheet with the back of a spoon or spatula.

6. Dehydrate it at 115°F for about 12 hours or until top of crackers is dry to the touch. Flip them over and dehydrate it about another 12 hours. Check on them every once in a while, to see if you think they're done or not. The longer you leave them in, the crunchier they are.

Recipe note: *If you don't have apple cider vinegar or fresh spices, make it with just the chia seeds, water and salt. The ACV and spices are just a tasty bonus. If your salt is currently restricted, make it with less salt or no salt. You'll still get chips with just the chia and water.*

You can also make this recipe with flaxseeds instead of chia seeds.

By Deanne Flickinger

I have been on a lifelong healing quest. Trying to figure out what to eat and not eat has been a journey. When I learned (how to eat) better, I ate better. And when I learned more, I would eat even better. After finding Dr. Goldner on YouTube in January 2023, I started hyper-nourishing. Within two weeks I could see to drive at night again! Today is 9/11/23 and I've just had my first exam in two years. I got even more good news. The astigmatism in my right eye has gotten better! And, that's one of those things that's not supposed to get better and progressively gets worse over time! Thank you, Dr. Goldner.

From The Author:

Thank you for purchasing this book. I hope it brings you great health and delicious meals!

I encourage you to continue your journey towards optimum health by continuing to learn as much as you can and be open to changing your habits and conquering food addictions.

While these recipes can drastically improve your health, you may still have residual symptoms or have less than optimal energy levels if your diet contains foods that cause diseases, you do not eat enough of the high nutrient foods, or drink enough water. Make sure you learn about the foods that make you sick and the food you need to restore your health in my book, Goodbye Lupus.

You can also struggle with recovery if you have other issues that interfere with recovery like poor sleep, food addictions, trauma, self-sabotage, or low moods. This is why I work without people on both foods and moods to help them get healthy as fast as possible. To learn more about the emotional and lifestyle issues that cause disease, make sure you read my book, Goodbye Autoimmune Disease.

If you are struggling with poor health and you want my help, I would love to help!

I give daily information and inspiration as well as regular live Q&A sessions for the public on my social media channels.

I also have online classes, articles, free recipes, and other resources available to help you recover your health on my websites.

If you want to work with me, I offer wellness appointments over zoom, and my Rapid Recovery programs to help with the daily support, accountability and the coaching you need to get this right and get as healthy as you can in the shortest time possible. When you work with me, I do everything I can to help you get the health you deserve.

Here is a list of resources and links to help you get healthy!

Social Media:

FACEBOOK: Facebook.com/DrGoldner

YOUTUBE: youtube.com/BrookeGoldnerMD

INSTAGRAM: @GoodbyeLupus

Websites:

GoodbyeLupus.com - For appointments, programs and free information.

SmoothieShred.com - For free smoothie recipes, videos about nutrition, wellness, and fitness.

I wish you the greatest health and happiness,

Brooke Goldner, M.D.

GoodbyeLupus.com

Citations:

1. Goldner, Brooke (2015). Goodbye Lupus, How A Medical Doctor Healed Herself Naturally With Supermarket Foods. ISBN-10 1516994027:

2. Goldner, Brooke (2019) Goodbye Autoimmune Disease, How To Prevent and Reverse Chronic Illness and Inflammatory Symptoms Using Supermarket Foods. ISBN-10 1729813909:

3. Siegel, RL, Wagle, NS, Cercek, A, Smith, RA, Jemal, A. Colorectal cancer statistics, 2023. *CA Cancer J Clin.* 2023; 1- 22. doi:10.3322/caac.21772

4. Thaddäus Tönnies, Ralph Brinks, Scott Isom, Dana Dabelea, Jasmin Divers, Elizabeth J. Mayer-Davis, Jean M. Lawrence, Catherine Pihoker, Lawrence Dolan, Angela D. Liese, Sharon H. Saydah, Ralph B. D'Agostino, Annika Hoyer, Giuseppina Imperatore; Projections of Type 1 and Type 2 Diabetes Burden in the U.S. Population Aged <20 Years Through 2060: The SEARCH for Diabetes in Youth Study. Diabetes Care 1 February 2023; 46 (2): 313–320.

5. Mori N, Shimazu T, Charvat H, Mutoh M, Sawada N, Iwasaki M, Yamaji T, Inoue M, Goto A, Takachi R, Ishihara J, Noda M, Iso H, Tsugane S; JPHC Study Group. Cruciferous vegetable intake and mortality in middle-aged adults: A prospective cohort study. Clin Nutr. 2019 Apr;38(2):631-643. doi: 10.1016/j.clnu.2018.04.012. Epub 2018 Apr 24. PMID: 29739681.

6. Campbell, Thomas (2016). The China study solution : the simple way to lose weight and reverse illness, using a whole-food, plant-based diet. Rodale Books. ISBN 9781623367572.

7. https://www.theguardian.com/science/2022/jan/08/global-spread-of-autoimmune-disease-blamed-on-western-diet

Made in the USA
Las Vegas, NV
30 March 2024